The Eye in Systemic Disease

Second edition

Colour Manuals in Ophthalmology

Retinal Detachment

by Jack J. Kanski

Uveitis

by Jack J. Kanski

Glaucoma

by Jack J. Kanski and
James A. McAllister

Contact Lenses in Ophthalmology

by Michael Wilson and
Elisabeth Millis

The Eye in Systemic Disease

Second edition

Jack J. Kanski, MD, MS, FRCS

Consultant Surgeon
Prince Charles Eye Unit,
King Edward VII Hospital, Windsor

Dafydd J. Thomas, MA, MD, FRCP

Consultant Neurologist
King Edward VII Hospital, Windsor,
St Mary's Hospital, London and The National
Hospital for Neurology and Neurosurgery,
London

Butterworth–Heinemann
London   Boston   Singapore
Sydney   Toronto   Wellington

PART OF REED INTERNATIONAL P.L.C.

First published 1986
Second edition 1990

Butterworth International Edition, 1990
ISBN 0-7506-1025-5

© **Butterworth–Heinemann Ltd, 1990**

British Library Cataloguing in Publication Data

Kanski, Jack J., Thomas, Dafydd J.
  The eye in systemic disease.
  2nd ed.
  1. Man. Diseases. syndromes
  I. Title
  616.047

ISBN 0-7506-1024-7

Library of Congress Cataloging-in-Publication Data

Kanski, Jack J., Thomas, Dafydd J.
    The eye in systemic disease/Jack J. Kanski.–2nd ed.
      p. cm.
    Includes bibliographical references.
    Includes index.
    ISBN 0-7506-1024-7 :
    1. Ocular manifestations of general diseases–Atlases.
    I. Title. [DNLM: 1. Eye Manifestations.   WW 475 K16e]
RE65.K36   1990
617.7–dc20   90-1944
                                         CIP

Composition by Genesis Typesetting, Laser Quay, Rochester, Kent
Printed in Scotland by Cambus Litho Ltd, Glasgow
Bound by Hartnolls Ltd, Bodmin, Cornwall

Preface to the second edition

The second edition of this book has undergone complete revision. Whilst the number of chapters has been reduced from eighteen to fifteen, the number of illustrations has been increased. In addition the systemic aspects of the diseases have been presented in greater detail and more emphasis has been placed on current methods of investigation such as CT and MR scanning.

Despite these modifications the main purpose of this book remains unchanged, that is to acquaint the general physician with a concise overview of the frequently complex relationships between the eye and medicine. For this reason detailed information of little or no interest to non-ophthalmologists which can be found in standard textbooks on ophthalmology has not been included.

We are greatly indebted to the following colleagues for reviewing the manuscript and for making many helpful suggestions: Dr Peter Mackie, Dr John Easton, Dr Ann Hall, Dr Robin Scott, Dr Michael Smith, Dr Stephen Dawson, Dr Ian White and Dr Teifi James. We would also like to thank Miss Daphne Bannister and Mrs Jane Tyler for taking many of the photographs and to Mr Terry Tarrant for the artwork.

J. J. K.
D. J. T.

Contents

1

Introduction

The main aim of this chapter is to familiarize the non-ophthalmologist with the various eye conditions that will be described in this book.

Conjunctivitis

Conjunctivitis is a very common, usually microbial, inflammation of the mucous membrane which lines the anterior sclera and the inside of the eyelids.

Causes

The most common causes are bacteria, chlamydia, and viruses. Occasional systemic associations include:

- Reiter's disease.
- Psoriatic arthritis.
- Wegener's granulomatosis.
- Cicatricial pemphigoid.
- Stevens–Johnson syndrome.
- Gonorrhoea.
- Crohn's disease.

Symptoms

Subacute onset of grittiness, usually bilateral, and a mucoid or serous discharge.

Signs

These include normal visual acuity, redness which is maximal in the lower fornices (Figure 1.1) and a variable amount of discharge.

Treatment

This is usually with topical antimicrobial agents.

Prognosis

This is excellent and, even without treatment, the vast majority resolve within 7–10 days.

Episcleritis

Episcleritis is a common non-microbial inflammation of the vascular connective tissue layer, which is located between the conjunctiva and the sclera. It typically affects one eye of a healthy middle-aged female.

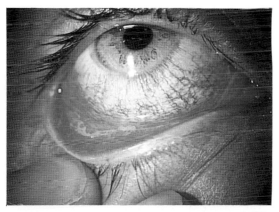

Figure 1.1 Acute conjunctivitis with maximal injection in the lower fornix

Causes

Most cases are idiopathic and unassociated with any systemic disease.

Symptoms

These are acute or subacute onset of mild unilateral discomfort and redness.

Signs

A localized red patch involving either the medial or the lateral aspects of the eye (Figure 1.2).

Treatment

Topical steroids may be helpful if started early.

Prognosis

This is excellent and most cases resolve within a few days but recurrences may occur.

Keratoconjunctivitis sicca

Keratoconjunctivitis sicca (KCS) is a common condition in which tear secretion by the lacrimal glands is reduced.

Causes

Pure KCS This is common and is characterized by involvement of the lacrimal gland alone.

Primary Sjögren's syndrome This is an autoimmune disease characterized by the frequent presence of rheumatoid factor, antinuclear antibodies and hypergammaglobulinaemia. Less common findings include antibodies to DNA, salivary duct tissue, smooth muscle and gastric parietal cells. Involvement of the salivary glands may cause a dry mouth (xerostomia), and the bronchial epithelium and the vagina may also be affected.

Secondary Sjögren's syndrome This is the presence of KCS in association with a systemic disorder such as:

- Rheumatoid arthritis.
- Psoriatic arthritis.
- Connective tissue disorder.
- Sarcoidosis.
- Crohn's disease.

Symptoms

These are chronic ocular irritation and a foreign body sensation.

Signs

Slit lamp biomicroscopy shows an absent or diminished lower lid tear meniscus, mucous threads in the tear film and corneal filaments. Rose bengal is a dye which shows up mucous threads and corneal filaments more clearly (Figure 1.3),

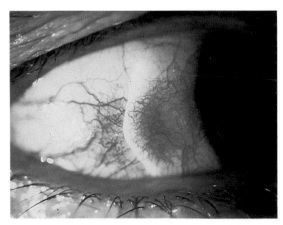

Figure 1.2 Localized area of injection in episcleritis (courtesy of Mr A. Shun-Shin)

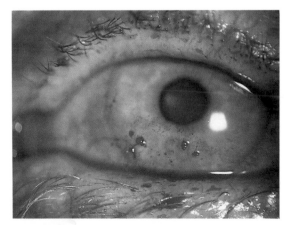

Figure 1.3 Mucous threads and corneal filaments in keratoconjunctivitis sicca stained with rose bengal

and also stains the bulbar conjunctiva in the form of two triangles with their bases at the limbus (Figure 1.4). The amount of tear secretion can also be determined by measuring the amount of moistening of a special strip of filter paper folded so that 5 mm of the strip lies within the conjunctival sac (*Schirmer's test*). A value of less than 5 mm in 5 minutes is indicative of KCS and values between 5 and 10 mm are borderline.

Treatment

Frequent instillation of artificial tears (e.g. hypromellose) is effective in most patients.

Prognosis

This is excellent although treatment may have to be continued indefinitely.

Keratitis

Keratitis is an inflammation of the cornea.

Causes

The most common causes are herpes simplex, herpes zoster, bacteria and hypersensitivity to staphylococcal exotoxins. Occasional systemic associations include:

- Rheumatoid arthritis.
- Connective tissue disorders
- Wegener's granulomatosis.
- Crohn's disease.
- Acne rosacea.
- Atopic eczema.
- Syphilis.

Symptoms

These are variable blurring of vision, watering, pain and photophobia.

Signs

Corneal haziness and ulceration are the two most common signs (Figure 1.5).

Treatment

Treatment is with topical antimicrobial agents and, in selected cases, steroids may also be indicated.

Prognosis

This is usually good provided treatment is started early.

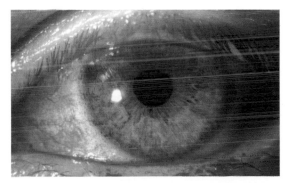

Figure 1.4 Conjunctival staining with rose bengal in keratoconjunctivitis sicca

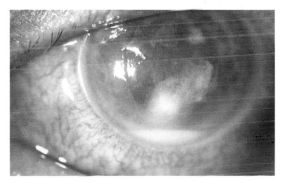

Figure 1.5 Severe bacterial keratitis with hypopyon

Scleritis

Scleritis is a very rare inflammation of the tough white outer collagenous layer of the eye.

Causes

The most common local cause is herpes zoster. The most frequent systemic associations include:

- Rheumatoid arthritis.
- Connective tissue disorders.
- Wegener's granulomatosis.

Symptoms and signs

For these see Chapter 4.

Treatment

Treatment is with systemic non-steroidal anti-inflammatory agents in mild cases, and steroids and/or cytotoxic agents in severe cases.

Prognosis

Many cases develop complications such as keratitis, cataract and glaucoma.

Anterior uveitis

Anterior uveitis (iridocyclitis) is an inflammation of the anterior part of the uveal tract which consists of the iris and ciliary body. The two main types are acute and chronic.

Acute anterior uveitis

Causes

Many cases are idiopathic. Systemic associations include:

- Ankylosing spondylitis.
- Reiter's syndrome.
- Psoriatic arthritis.
- Behçet's disease.
- Sarcoidosis.
- Syphilis.
- Crohn's disease.
- Ulcerative colitis.

Symptoms

These are subacute onset of unilateral photophobia, pain, redness, decreased vision and watering.

Signs

These are a small pupil, circumcorneal 'ciliary' injection, which has a violaceous hue (Figure 1.6), and inflammatory cells in the aqueous humour (Figure 1.7), which can be detected only with a special microscope called a slit lamp. In very severe cases a fibrinous exudate develops in the aqueous (Figure 1.8) and the inflammatory cells may form a white fluid level in the bottom of the anterior chamber called a hypopyon (see Figure 4.25).

Treatment

This is with topical steroids to suppress the inflammation and mydriatics to prevent the

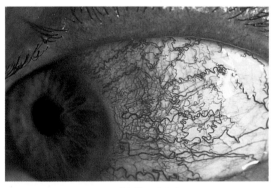

Figure 1.6 Circumcorneal (ciliary) injection in acute iritis

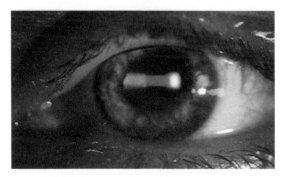

Figure 1.7 Acute iritis with aqueous cells and flare as seen with the slit lamp microscope

formation of adhesions between the iris and lens called posterior synechiae (Figure 1.9).

Prognosis

This is usually good provided treatment is instituted early. Most cases last less than 6 weeks although recurrences are common.

Chronic anterior uveitis

Chronic anterior uveitis is less common than the acute type. It frequently persists for several months and sometimes for years.

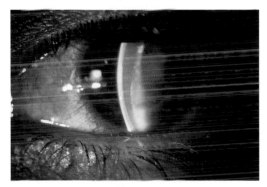

Figure 1.8 Fibrinous exudate in the aqueous in very severe acute iritis associated with ankylosing spondylitis

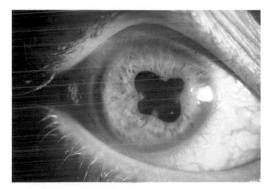

Figure 1.9 Irregular pupil due to adhesions between the iris and lens (posterior synechiae) following a severe attack of acute iritis

Causes

Some cases are idiopathic. Systemic associations include:

- Sarcoidosis.
- Tuberculosis.
- Juvenile chronic arthritis.
- Syphilis.
- Whipple's disease.

Symptoms

These may be minimal despite severe inflammation. Patients may report slight blurring of vision and mild redness.

Signs

These are similar to the acute type, although the eye is not usually red and the condition is frequently bilateral.

Treatment

Treatment is similar to the acute type although the response may be less satisfactory.

Prognosis

This is less good than in the acute type. The inflammation may persist for many months and even years and give rise to complications such as glaucoma, band keratopthy and cataract (see Figure 4.20)

Cataract

A cataract is an opacity in the crystalline lens of the eye.

Causes

Old age is by far the most common cause. Other causes include:

- Trauma and irradiation.
- Inherited.
- Chronic anterior uveitis.
- Steroids.
- Diabetes.

Symptoms

There is usually a gradual impairment of vision.

Signs

A lens opacity can be detected by observing the red reflex with an ophthalmoscope held about 30 cm from the patient's eye (Figure 1.10).

Treatment

Treatment is surgical.

Prognosis

This is excellent in the vast majority.

Posterior uveitis

Posterior uveitis is an inflammation of the choroid and/or retina. According to the site of primary involvement it is subdivided into retinitis, choroiditis and retinochoroiditis.

Causes

In the UK the most common cause is reactivation of congenital toxoplasmosis. Systemic associations include:

- Behçet's disease.
- Sarcoidosis.
- Tuberculosis.
- AIDS.
- Syphilis.
- Crohn's disease.
- Whipple's disease.
- Reticulum cell sarcoma.

Signs

These vary according to the type.

- Vitritis is characterized by cells in the vitreous. It is responsible for symptoms of vitreous floaters and, if severe, it impairs visualization of the fundus.
- Active retinochoroiditis is characterized by white cloudy patches with indistinct outlines (Figure 1.11).

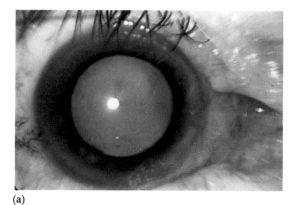

(a)

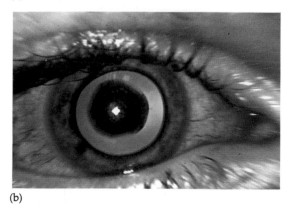

(b)

Figure 1.10 (a) Normal red reflex; (b) red reflex in an eye with a central lens opacity

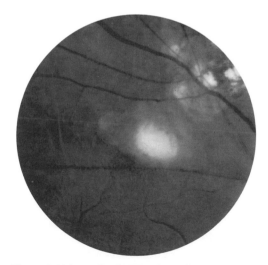

Figure 1.11 Acute focal retinochoroiditis due to toxoplasmosis – note old inactive lesions

- Inactive retinochoroiditis appears as white well-defined areas of chorioretinal atrophy with pigmented borders. The retinal blood vessels pass over the lesions undisturbed (Figure 1.12).
- Vasculitis may involve the retinal veins (periphlebitis) or, less commonly, the arterioles. Active periphlebitis is characterized by a fluffy white haziness surrounding the blood column (see Figure 7.9).

Treatment

This varies according to the cause and includes systemic antimicrobial agents, steroids and cytotoxic agents.

Prognosis

This varies according to the cause and location of the inflammatory focus. Lesions involving the fovea have a poor prognosis.

Vascular disorders of the fundus

Haemorrhages

- Flame-shaped haemorrhages are located in the superficial nerve fibre layer of the retina. They may occur in hypertension, papilloedema and retinal vein occlusion (see Figures 3.6 and 3.7).
- Dot and blot haemorrhages lie deep in the plexiform or inner nuclear layers of the retina. They typically occur in background diabetic retinopathy (see Figure 2.26).
- Dark blot haemorrhages involve the entire thickness of the retina and are frequently indicative of severe retinal ischaemia.
- Roth's spots are haemorrhages with white centres which may occur in endocarditis and various haematological diseases (see Figure 11.1).

Cotton-wool spots

These were formerly referred to as soft exudates. They lie in the nerve fibre layer of the retina and appear as fluffy white patches most commonly at the posterior pole (Figure 1.13). Cotton-wool spots

are associated with many conditions that cause retinal ischaemia such as:

- Retinal vein occlusion.
- Preproliferative diabetic retinopathy.
- Hypertensive retinopathy.
- Collagen vascular disorders.
- AIDS.
- Papilloedema.
- Blood hyperviscosity.

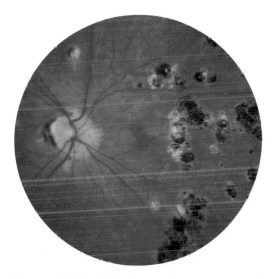

Figure 1.12 Old multifocal retinochoroiditis

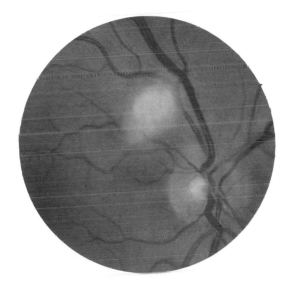

Figure 1.13 Large cotton-wool spot

Hard exudates

These form in areas of chronic focal vascular leakage and consist of deposits of lipids and lipoproteins. Hard exudates lie deep in the retina and appear as yellowish lesions with well-demarcated borders.

- In background diabetic retinopathy, the hard exudates frequently form circinate rings (see Figure 2.30).
- In papilloedema and hypertensive retinopathy, they form a star figure centred at the fovea (macular star) (Figure 1.14).

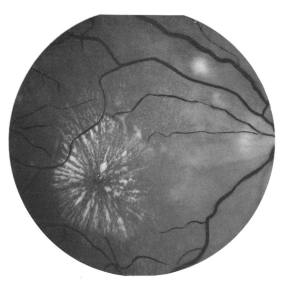

Figure 1.14 Macular star in hypertensive retinopathy – also a small cotton-wool spot near the superotemporal arcade (courtesy of Dr P. Malleson)

Ischaemic optic neuropathy

Cause

This is caused by infarction of the anterior part of the optic nerve by occlusion of the posterior ciliary arteries. The majority of patients are elderly with no obvious underlying disease except presumed atheroma and possibly mild hypertension or diabetes. Systemic associations include:

- Giant cell arteritis.
- Collagen vascular disorders.
- Wegener's granulomatosis.

Symptoms

These are acute unilateral visual loss.

Signs

These are pale swelling of the optic disc which may be associated with a few flame-shaped haemorrhages (see Figure 3.11).

Treatment

Treatment is with systemic steroids if associated with a systemic disease.

Prognosis

This is poor, especially in giant cell arteritis.

2

Endocrine disorders

Thyroid dysfunction

Basic thyroid physiology

- Two hormones secreted by the thyroid gland are *thyroxine* (T_4) and *triiodthyronine* (T_3) (Figure 2.1). The enzymatic reactions in which iodine is trapped and incorporated into these two hormones are under the control of the anterior pituitary via the thyroid-stimulating hormone (TSH). The anterior pituitary is, in turn, influenced by the hypothalamus by thyrotrophin-releasing hormone (TRH). Both the anterior pituitary and the hypothalamus are under feedback control so that secretion varies inversely with the levels of circulating T_3 and T_4.
- In the plasma over 99.95% of both T_3 and T_4 are bound to protein and only 0.05% of both hormones exists in an unbound state or free form. However, despite their exceedingly low concentrations, these free fractions are very important because they diffuse out of the circulation and enter cells where they exert their biological actions. T_3 is thought to be as important as T_4 in total metabolic activity despite the fact that its concentration is very much lower. Occasionally T_3 thyrotoxicosis occurs in the presence of a normal T_4.
- Thyroid function tests include: (1) total serum T_3 and T_4, (2) serum free T_3 and T_4, (3) serum TSH, (4) TRH stress test and (5) thyroid antibodies. Most laboratories now measure TSH with a highly sensitive immunoradiometric assay as a screening test for both hypo- and hyperthyroid states. It is now rarely necessary to perform a TRH test.

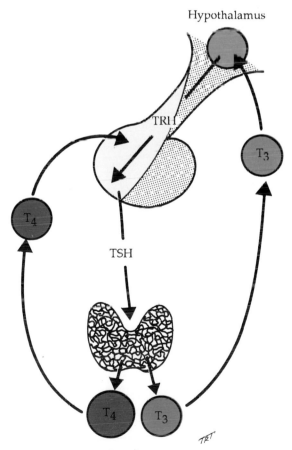

Figure 2.1 Thyroid physiology

9

Hyperthyroidism

Classification

Graves' disease   This is a common autoimmune disease caused by excess secretion of thyroid hormones by the entire thyroid gland. It typically affects females and is the most frequent cause of hyperthyroidism (thyrotoxicosis).

Toxic nodular goitre   This is characterized by excess secretion of thyroid hormones by single or multiple thyroid nodules. It is less common than Graves' disease and it usually occurs in an older age group.

Subacute thyroiditis   This may cause transient hyperthyroidism.

Factitious hyperthyroidism   This is caused by excessive ingestion of thyroid hormones.

Clinical features

Presentation

- Weight loss despite increased appetite and food intake.
- Increased bowel frequency.
- Sweating and heat intolerance.
- Nervousness, irritability, palpitation, weakness, fatigue and tremor.

Signs

External

- Warm and sweaty skin, fine silky hair, onycholysis affecting the finger nails, especially the ring fingers (Plummer's nails).
- Pretibial myxoedema (infiltrative dermopathy) (Figure 2.2) and clubbing of the finger nails (thyroid acropathy) (Figure 2.3) may be present in Graves' disease.
- Diffuse thyroid enlargement in Graves' disease may be associated with a bruit.
- One or more nodules may be palpable in patients with nodular goitre.

Cardiovascular

- Sinus tachycardia, wide pulse pressure and high output cardiac failure.
- Arrhythmias (atrial fibrillation and premature ventricular beats).

Central nervous system

- Fine tremor and brisk tendon reflexes.
- Muscle weakness due to associated proximal myopathy is common.
- Myasthenic features are occasionally seen.

Treatment

The options for control are:

- Oral antithyroid drugs (e.g. carbimazole).
- Surgical partial thyroidectomy.

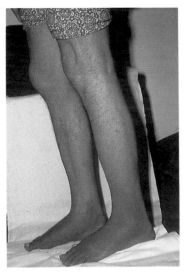

Figure 2.2 Pretibial myxoedema

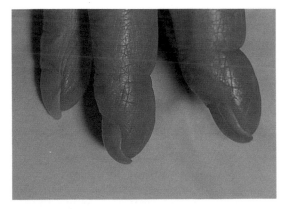

Figure 2.3 Thyroid acropathy

- Radioactive iodine therapy.
- β-Blockers are useful for symptomatic relief of sweating, tachycardia and tremor.

In patients with thyrotoxicosis and ophthalmopathy, it is generally advisable to change thyroid status gently.

Thyroid ophthalmopathy

Association with hyperthyroidism

Sometimes thyroid ophthalmopathy may exist without any clinical or biochemical evidence of thyroid dysfunction. More frequently there are some systemic features, but they may follow a completely different clinical course from ocular involvement. When the eye signs of Graves' disease occur in a patient who is not clinically hyperthyroid, the condition is referred to as euthyroid or ophthalmic Graves' disease. This is the form which is most frequently encountered by ophthalmologists. In patients with Graves' disease the eye signs may precede, coincide with or follow the hyperthyroidism. In general the ocular features of Graves' disease and ophthalmic euthyroid Graves' disease are similar, although they tend to be more asymmetrical in the latter (Figure 2.4).

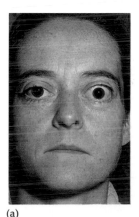
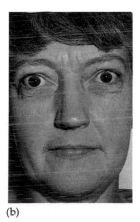

(a)   (b)

Figure 2.4 Thyroid ophthalmopathy. (a) Asymmetrical features in ophthalmic (euthyroid) Graves' disease; (b) symmetrical signs in Graves' disease

Classification

- Eyelid signs.
- Infiltrative ophthalmopathy:
    Soft tissue involvement.
    Proptosis.
    Optic neuropathy.
    Restrictive myopathy.

Eyelid signs

Lid retraction (Dalrymple's sign) Retraction of both the upper and lower lids is one of the cardinal signs of Graves' disease and is responsible for both functional and cosmetic problems. In many patients there is both true lid retraction as well as pseudo-lid retraction due to associated proptosis.

Mechanisms Although the phenomenon of lid retraction is incompletely understood, a combination of the following factors is responsible:

- Over-action of Müller's muscle due to sympathetic over-stimulation.
- Over-action of the superior rectus and levator muscles secondary to restrictive myopathy of the inferior rectus muscle.
- Restrictive myopathy of the levator muscle itself.

Clinical features In the normal eye the upper eyelid covers about 2 mm of the superior part of the cornea (Figure 2.5a). Lid retraction is recognized by elevation of the upper lid so that its margin is either level with or above the superior limbus, allowing sclera to be visible (Figure 2.5b).

Lid lag (Von Graefe's sign) This is characterized by the retarded descent of the upper lid on looking down (Figure 2.6). When gaze is changed from down to up, the globe then lags behind the upper lid.

Miscellaneous lid signs

- Staring and frightened appearance which is particularly marked on attentive fixation (Kocher's sign) (Figure 2.7).
- Infrequent blinking.
- Marked fine tremor on lid closure.
- Jerky movements on lid opening.

In about 50% of patients lid retraction improves with the passage of time and its severity is usually improved by treatment of the hyperthyroidism.

Differential diagnosis   Other causes of lid retraction include:

- Aberrant regeneration of the third nerve (see Chapter 6).
- Unilateral ptosis with contralateral over-action of the levator (e.g. myasthenia).
- Collier's sign of the dorsal midbrain (Parinaud's syndrome) (see Chapter 6).
- Familial periodic paralysis.

Infiltrative ophthalmopathy

Pathogenesis   A humoral agent (IgG antibody) is probably responsible for the following changes (Figure 2.8):

- Enlargement of extraocular muscles associated with an increase in glycosaminoglycans and oedema in the extracellular tissues.
- Round cell infiltration of interstitial tissues, and

subsequent degeneration of muscle fibres, eventually leads to fibrosis which exerts a tethering effect on the involved muscle and results in restrictive myopathy.

- Proliferation of orbital fat and connective tissue is associated with retention of fluid, accumulation of glycosaminoglycans and round cell infiltration.

The above factors cause an increase in the size of intraorbital contents and a secondary elevation of intraorbital pressure, which may itself cause further fluid retention within the orbit.

Soft tissue involvement

- Conjunctival injection is a sensitive sign of disease activity. An intense focal hyperaemia may be seen outlining and overlying the tendons of the horizontal rectus muscles (Figure 2.9).

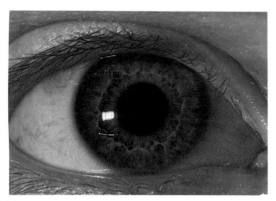

(a)

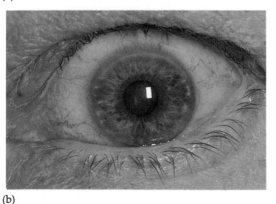

(b)

Figure 2.5 (a) Normal position of the upper eyelid hiding the superior part of the cornea; (b) exposure of sclera due to lid retraction

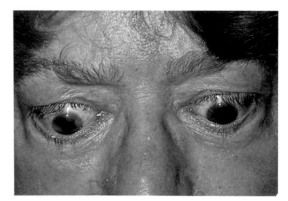

Figure 2.6 Lid lag on downgaze (Von Graefe's sign)

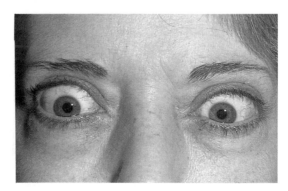

Figure 2.7 Staring and frightened appearance (Kocher's sign)

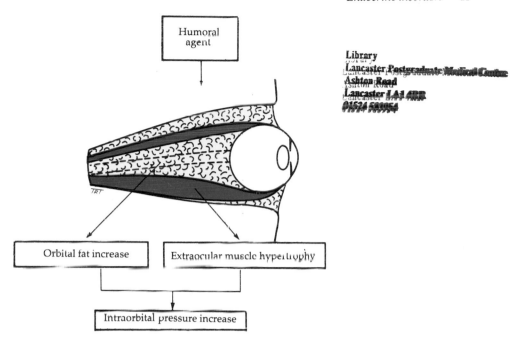

Figure 2.8 Postulated pathogenesis of infiltrative thyroid ophthalmopathy

- Chemosis refers to oedema of the conjunctiva and caruncle. If minimal it is manifest as a small fold of redundant conjunctiva overhanging the lower eyelid. If severe the conjunctiva prolapses over the lower lid (Figure 2.10).
- Superior limbic keratoconjunctivitis is characterized by papillary hypertrophy of the upper tarsal plate, and hyperaemia and thickening of the superior bulbar conjunctiva (Figure 2.11).

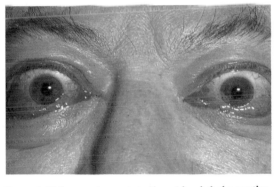

Figure 2.10 Severe chemosis in thyroid ophthalmopathy

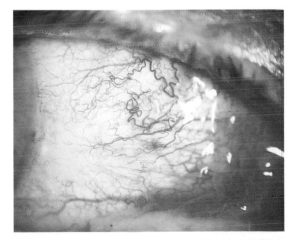

Figure 2.9 Conjunctival injection overlying a medial rectus muscle

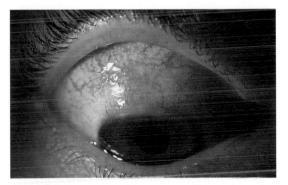

Figure 2.11 Injection of the superior bulbar conjunctiva due to superior limbic keratoconjunctivitis

Proptosis

Measurement   The normal distance between the apex of the cornea and the lateral orbital rim is 20 mm. Any measurement of 21 mm or more is regarded as being abnormal and indicative of proptosis, which is defined as a forward protrusion of the globe. Proptosis is best detected by examining the patient from above (Figure 2.12). The amount of proptosis can be measured either with a Hertel exophthalmometer (Figure 2.13) or a plastic rule resting on bone at the outer canthus (Figure 2.14).

Clinical features   In thyroid ophthalmopathy proptosis is very common and it may be unilateral, bilateral and asymmetrical. It may be self-limiting, is uninfluenced by the treatment of the hyperthyroidism and it persists in about 70% of patients. It is useful to think of proptosis as being a safety mechanism which protects the optic nerve from the potentially dangerous effects of raised intra-orbital pressure. However, in some patients with a strong orbital septum the intraorbital pressure may rise to dangerous levels without causing proptosis.

Differential diagnosis   Whilst thyroid ophthalmopathy is the most common cause of both unilateral and bilateral proptosis in adults the following causes should also be considered.

Pseudoproptosis due to:

- Ipsilateral lid retraction.
- Ipsilateral enlargement of the globe resulting from very severe myopia (Figure 2.15) or buphthalmos due to congenital glaucoma.
- Ipsilateral shallow orbit (e.g. craniofacial dysostosis, facial and skull asymmetry).
- Contralateral enophthalmos.

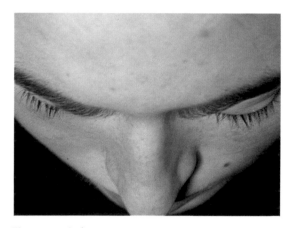

Figure 2.12 Left proptosis seen from above

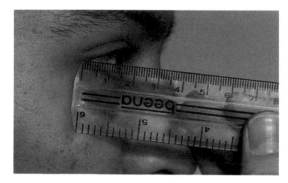

Figure 2.14 Measurement of amount of proptosis with a plastic rule

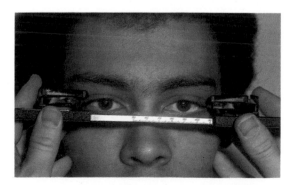

Figure 2.13 Measurement of amount of proptosis with a Hertel exophthalmometer

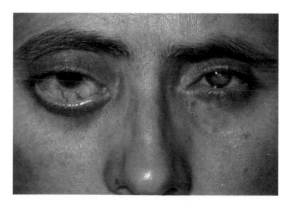

Figure 2.15 Right pseudoproptosis due to a combination of a large right eye from high myopia and a small shrunken left eye

Other common causes of true proptosis in adults are:

- Orbital tumours.
- Orbital pseudotumours.
- Vascular anomalies.

Optic neuropathy   This is a rare but potentially very serious complication that requires immediate treatment. It has an insidious onset and is easy to miss, because it may occur in the absence of significant proptosis and in eyes with normal visual acuity. Its presence may also be masked by other symptoms.

Pathogenesis   The pathogenesis of optic neuropathy has been ascribed to many different causes. It seems likely that apical orbital crowding by enlarged extraocular muscles is an important factor (Figures 2.16 and 2.17).

Visual function   The most sensitive symptoms of early optic nerve dysfunction are a greying of vision or desaturation of colours. Patients rarely volunteer the latter unless specifically questioned. Visual acuity is reduced in 50% of cases. In order to detect early optic neuropathy, patients should be encouraged to monitor periodically their own vision at home by alternately occluding each eye and reading small print as well as assessing the intensity of colours on a television screen.

Visual fields   About 60% of patients have visual field abnormalities which include: increased size of the blind spot, paracentral scotomata, nerve fibre bundle defects, central or paracentral scotomata and generalized constriction.

Signs

- The optic nerve head in 50% of patients with optic neuropathy is normal, in 25% it is elevated and hyperaemic (Figure 2.18), and in 25% it is pale.
- A relative afferent pupillary conduction defect is common.

Restrictive myopathy   The possibility of thyroid eye disease should be suspected in all adults who complain of double vision, especially if the two

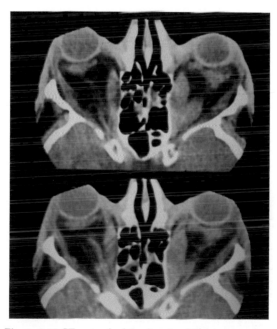

Figure 2.16 CT scan of orbits showing large extraocular muscles in thyroid ophthalmopathy (courtesy of Mr P. Rosen)

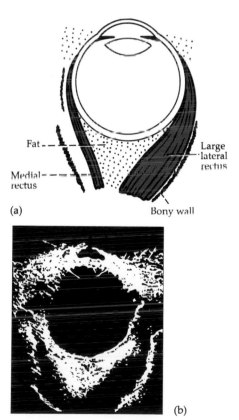

(a)

(b)

Figure 2.17 (a) Large lateral rectus muscle in thyroid ophthalmopathy; (b) appearance on B-scan ultrasonography

images are separated vertically. In order of frequency, defects of ocular motility caused by fibrotic contactions of extraocular muscles are:

- Inferior rectus contraction causing defective elevation which mimics a superior rectus palsy – the most common (Figure 2.19).
- Medial rectus contraction causing defective abduction which mimics a sixth nerve palsy (Figure 2.20).
- Superior rectus contraction causing defective depression which mimics an inferior rectus palsy.
- Lateral rectus contraction causing defective adduction – the least common.

Treatment of thyroid ophthalmopathy

Non-specific

- Reassurance that, in many cases, involvement is relatively mild and that the condition resolves spontaneously within several months or a few years and is merely a nuisance. All that these patients require is examination every 6 months to ensure that they are not developing any vision-threatening complications.
- Head elevation during sleep by blocks under the head of the bed and extra pillows may reduce the severity of periorbital oedema.

- Taping of eyelids at night to protect the cornea in patients with exposure keratopathy.
- Prismatic spectacles may be useful in controlling mild diplopia.
- Diuretics such as cyclopenthiazide (Navidrex-K) 0.5 mg at bedtime may be useful in reducing the severity of morning periorbital oedema.

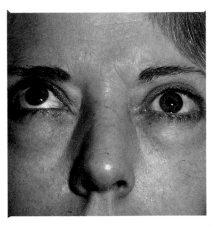

Figure 2.19 Defective elevation of left eye due to restrictive thyroid myopathy of the left inferior rectus muscle

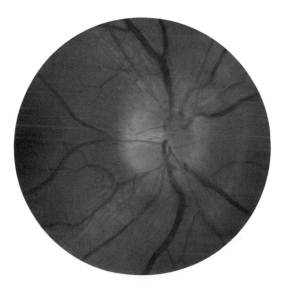

Figure 2.18 Moderate disc swelling in dysthyroid optic neuropathy

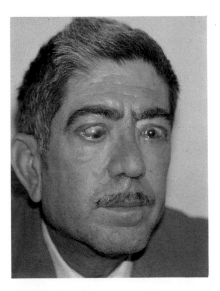

Figure 2.20 Gross convergent strabismus due to bilateral contracture of the medial rectus muscles simulating bilateral sixth nerve palsies (courtesy of Mr B. Mathalone)

Ocular lubricants Chronic ocular irritation in patients with thyroid ophthalmopathy may be caused by conjunctival inflammation, corneal exposure, dry eyes due to infiltration of the lacrimal glands by inflammatory cells, and superior limbic keratoconjunctivitis. Lubricants in the form of artificial tears during the day and ointment at bedtime are useful in obtaining symptomatic relief.

Systemic steroids

Indications Systemic steroid therapy is indicated for optic neuropathy and during the *early* course of the disease in patients with severe chemosis, proptosis and pain (Figure 2.21). Steroid therapy, however, has no effect on the severity of either restrictive ocular myopathy or lid retraction, and it is of no value in long-standing cases.

Administration An initial dose of enteric-coated prednisolone 80–100 mg/day should be administered and a favourable response expected within 48 hours with reduction of discomfort, chemosis and periorbital oedema. The dose should then be tapered by 5 mg every fifth day. A maximal response is usually achieved within 2–8 weeks. If possible, steroid therapy should be terminated after 3 months. Prolonged steroid administration should be reserved only for the few patients who are unresponsive to other forms of therapy. The benefits of azathioprine and cyclophosphamide either alone or as steroid-sparing agents are uncertain.

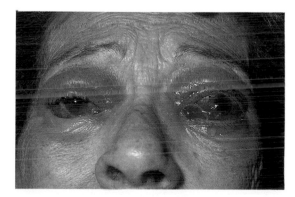

Figure 2.21 Extremely severe dysthyroid ophthalmopathy with exposure keratopathy of the left eye

Radiotherapy

Indications The indications for radiotherapy are essentially the same as for steroid therapy. It is mainly reserved for patients who:

* Have systemic contraindications to steroids.
* Refuse steroids.
* Develop serious steroid side effects.
* Are steroid resistant.

Administration The dose is 20 Gy to the posterior orbit given over a 10-day period. A positive response is usually evident within 6 weeks with maximal improvement evident by 4 months. Patients who are unresponsive to steroids may benefit from radiotherapy which, just like steroid therapy, does not influence the degree of restrictive ocular myopathy or lid retraction. Potential complications of radiotherapy include: cataract formation, keratitis, localized oedema and mild loss of hair.

Orbital decompression

Indications In general decompression of the orbit should only be considered when non-invasive methods (i.e. systemic steroids, radiotherapy) have been tried and been proved ineffective. The three main indications are:

1. Severe exposure keratopathy secondary to proptosis and lid retraction.
2. Optic neuropathy with imminent danger of permanent visual damage.
3. Cosmetically unacceptable proptosis. Because of the potential complications of surgical decompression, this applies only to patients in whom the proptosis has been stable for at least 9 months.

Methods

* One-wall decompression involving either the medial or lateral walls.
* Two-wall (antral–ethmoidal) decompression (Figure 2.22) which is the most popular.
* Three-wall decompression in which the lateral wall is also removed.
* Four-wall decompression in which a part of the sphenoid bone at the apex of the orbit and the lateral half of the roof are also removed.

Surgery on extraocular muscles   Operation on the extraocular muscles for restrictive myopathy should only be performed when the angle of deviation has been stable for at least 6 months. The goals of surgery are to achieve binocular single vision in the primary position of gaze and when reading.

Surgery on eyelids

- Joining together of the upper and lower eyelids (tarsorrhaphy) is indicated for uncontrolled exposure keratopathy.
- Surgery to weaken Müller's muscle for patients with severe lid retraction (Figure 2.23).
- Removal of excess fatty tissue and redundant skin from around the eyelids (blepharoplasty).

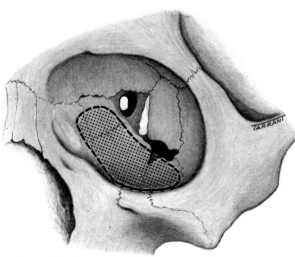

Figure 2.22 Two-wall orbital decompression

Diabetes mellitus

Definition

Diabetes mellitus is an extremely common disease characterized by sustained hyperglycaemia secondary to lack, or diminished efficacy, of endogenous insulin. The two main types are: (1) *insulin-dependent* (type 1, juvenile-onset) and (2) *non-insulin-dependent* (type 2, maturity-onset).

Diagnostic tests

- Urinalysis for glucose and ketones.
- Random blood glucose over 11 mmol/l is suggestive.
- Fasting blood glucose persistently over 7.2 mmol/l is virtually diagnostic.
- Glucose tolerance test may be useful in borderline cases.

Systemic features

Presentation

- Polyuria, polydipsia and nocturia are the most common presenting features of hyperglycaemia.
- Weight loss and infections of the skin, vulva and urinary tract are also frequent.
- Incidental finding.

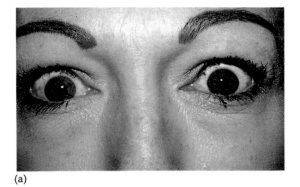
(a)

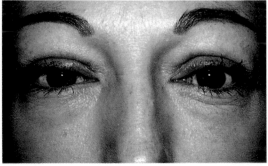
(b)

Figure 2.23 (a) Severe bilateral lid retraction – preoperative appearance; (b) appearance following bilateral recession of the levator and Müller's muscles

Acute complications

- Diabetic ketoacidosis in insulin-dependent diabetics (IDDs).
- Hypoglycaemic coma due to insulin excess, excessive physical activity and sulphonylureas.
- Hyperosmolar non-ketotic coma typically affects elderly non-insulin-dependent diabetics (NIDDs).

Chronic complications

Nephropathy This has multiple causes (e.g. papillary necrosis, chronic interstitial nephritis). The lesion specific for diabetes is intracapillary glomerulosclerosis (Kimmelstiel–Wilson syndrome) characterized by initial proteinuria, which may progress to the nephrotic syndrome and then to chronic renal failure.

Accelerated atherosclerosis

- Coronary artery disease is more common in diabetics.
- Peripheral vascular disease of the lower limbs with poorly healing ulcers, gangrene and eventual amputation.

Neuropathy

- Peripheral sensory neuropathy which may be painful but is often asymptomatic. In advanced cases, a symmetrical glove and stocking sensory disturbance is found and in mild cases just the toes are numb.
- Autonomic neuropathy is characterized by postural hypotension, nocturnal diarrhoea, gustatory sweating, impotence and abnormal bladder function.
- Radiculopathy characterized by pain involving a single nerve root or a single cranial nerve possibly as a result of ischaemic infarction.
- Mononeuritis multiplex where several peripheral nerves are involved, especially the median, ulnar and lateral popliteal.

Treatment

The goals of treatment of diabetes are to control symptoms and to prevent acute and chronic complications by the following measures:

- Diet involving the regulation and timing of carbohydrate intake.
- Oral hypoglycaemic agents in NIDDs not controlled by diet alone.
- Insulin is indicated in IDDs and in some NIDDs in whom satisfactory control is not obtained by other measures.

Ocular complications

Classification

- Diabetic retinopathy:
    Background.
    Maculopathy.
    Preproliferative.
    Proliferative.
    Advanced diabetic eye disease.
- Cataract:
    Accelerated senile.
    True diabetic.
- Ocular motor nerve palsies.
- Abnormal pupillary reactions.
- Changes in refraction.

Diabetic retinopathy (DR)

Prevalence

Overall prevalence of retinopathy in diabetic patients is about 25%. In NIDDs the prevalence is 20% and in IDDs it is about 40%.

Risk factors

Duration of diabetes The incidence of diabetic retinopathy (DR) is closely related to the duration of diabetes. In patients diagnosed as having diabetes prior to the age of 30 years, the incidence of DR is 50% after 10 years and 90% after 30 years. It is extremely rare for DR to develop within 5 years of the onset of diabetes, but about 5% of NIDDs have background DR at presentation.

Control of diabetes Although good control will not prevent DR, it may retard its development by a few years. Conversely, poorly controlled patients may develop DR sooner than well-controlled patients. The growing conviction that complications of diabetes are linked to poor metabolic control has led to aggressive efforts to normalize metabolism. However, in some patients a worsening of retinopathy has been observed during the first few months to one year of improved blood glucose control, whether achieved by continuous subcutaneous infusion with insulin pumps or by multiple injections.

Miscellaneous   The following may have an adverse effect on DR:

- Pregnancy.
- Hypertension
- Renal disease.
- Anaemia.

When to screen

Insulin-dependent diabetics

- Newly diagnosed: no need to screen for at least 5 years.
- Five to 10 years after the initial diagnosis: screen annually.
- Over 10 years after the initial diagnosis: screen every 6 months.

Non-insulin-dependent diabetics

- Screen at least annually.

Background diabetic retinopathy

Clinical features   Background DR is by far the most common type. It is caused by microvascular leakage into the retina. In the absence of maculopathy it is asymptomatic. The signs are the following:

- Microaneurysms are the earliest lesions consisting of small red dots which are usually located at the posterior pole temporal to the fovea (Figure 2.24).
- Dot and blot haemorrhages are common and are located within the compact deep retinal layers. Small dot haemorrhages may be difficult to differentiate from microaneurysms (Figure 2.25).
- Hard exudates are more advanced lesions which are frequently located in a circinate pattern peripheral to areas of chronic intraretinal leakage (Figures 2.26 and 2.27).
- Diffuse retinal oedema causes retinal thickening which is difficult to detect, particularly by the non-expert.

Management

- Treat associated hypertension, anaemia or renal failure.
- Annual fundus examination.

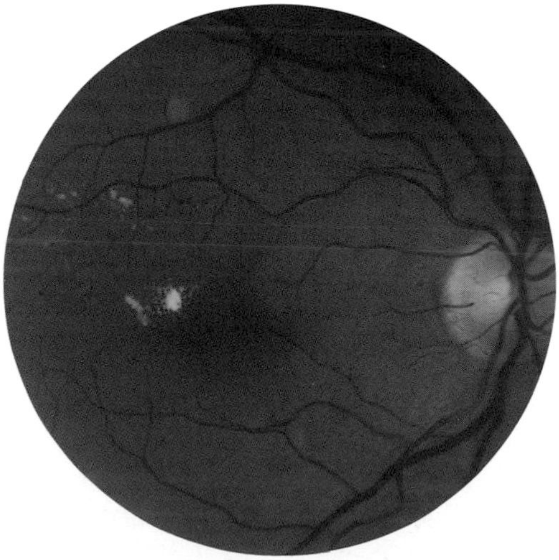

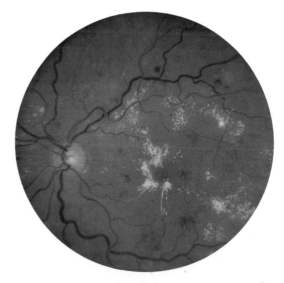

Figure 2.24 Mild background diabetic retinopathy with microaneurysms superotemporal to the fovea and a few hard exudates; visual acuity is normal

Figure 2.25 Moderate background diabetic retinopathy with scattered haemorrhages and hard exudates very near to the fovea; visual acuity is normal

Diabetic maculopathy

Clinical features Maculopathy is the most common cause of visual impairment in patients with DR and is more frequent in NIDDs. It is caused by involvement of the fovea by oedema and/or hard exudates.

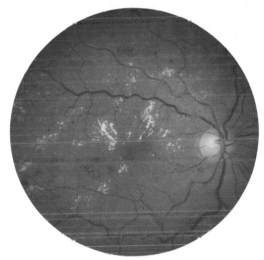

Figure 2.26 Severe background diabetic retinopathy with haemorrhages and many scattered hard exudates; visual acuity is normal

- Symptoms are a gradual impairment of central vision, such as difficulty in reading small print or seeing road signs.
- Signs consist of background DR associated with involvement of fovea by oedema or hard exudates (Figure 2.28).

Management Refer to an ophthalmologist (non-urgent) because laser photocoagulation will stablize (but seldom improve) visual acuity in about 50% of cases.

Preproliferative diabetic retinopathy

Clinical features This uncommon type of DR is caused by retinal hypoxia. It is asymptomatic in the absence of maculopathy. The signs are (Figure 2.29):

- Cotton-wool spots due to capillary occlusion in the nerve fibre layers.
- Intraretinal microvascular abnormalities (IRMAs) which are thought to represent intra-retinal neovascularization.
- Venous changes consisting of dilatation, beading, looping and sausage-like segmentation.
- Arteriolar narrowing which may resemble a branch retinal artery occlusion.
- Large, dark blot haemorrhages which represent haemorrhagic infarcts.

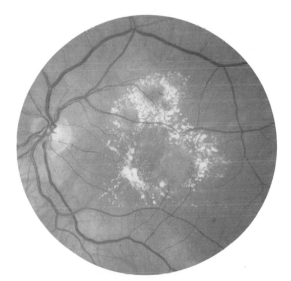

Figure 2.27 Severe background diabetic retinopathy with large rings of hard exudates

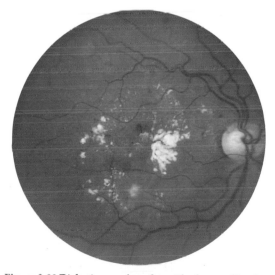

Figure 2.28 Diabetic maculopathy with plaque of hard exudate at the fovea; visual acuity is 6/36

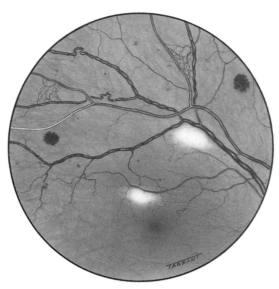

Figure 2.29 Composite illustration showing the various features of preproliferative diabetic retinopathy

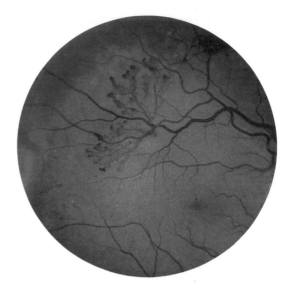

Figure 2.31 Proliferative diabetic retinopathy with moderate flat retinal new vessels

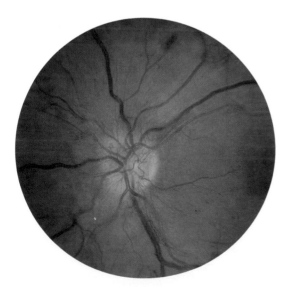

Figure 2.30 Proliferative diabetic retinopathy with moderate flat disc new vessels

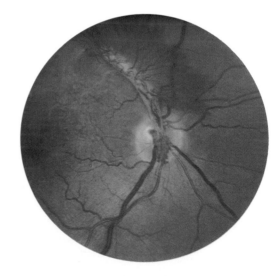

Figure 2.32 Severe proliferative diabetic retinopathy with fibrovascular proliferation extending from the disc along the superotemporal arcade

Management Although treatment by laser is usually unnecessary, refer to an ophthalmologist (semi-urgent) because a close follow-up is required so that proliferative changes can be detected and treated early.

Proliferative diabetic retinopathy

Clinical features This uncommon type typically affects IDDs. It is caused by severe retinal hypoxia.

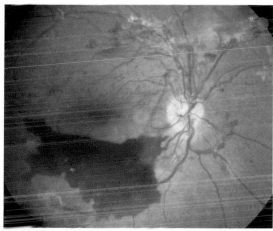

(a)

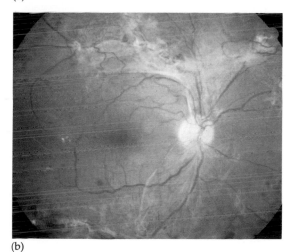

(b)

Figure 2.33 (a) Severe proliferative diabetic retinopathy with extensive neovascularization involving the superotemporal arcade and inferior preretinal haemorrhage; (b) regression of new vessels following laser photocoagulation. Note the residual avascular fibrous tissue

It is asymptomatic in the absence of complications. The signs include:

- Early signs are neovascularization on the disc (Figure 2.30) or away from the disc (Figure 2.31). Initially the new vessels are bare and flat and may be easily missed on cursory examination.
- Late signs are elevated new vessels which may be associated with a white fibrous component and which are easier to detect (Figure 2.32).

Management All patients with proliferative disease should be referred (urgent) to an ophthalmologist because they will require laser treatment (Figures 2.33 and 2.34).

Advanced diabetic eye disease

Clinical features This is now rare provided proliferative DR is treated adequately. Early symptoms are a sudden onset of floaters and blurred vision due to vitreous haemorrhage. Later the eye becomes blind due to a combination of the following:

- Persistent dense vitreous haemorrhage.
- Tractional retinal detachment (Figure 2.35).
- Neovascular glaucoma associated with the formation of new blood vessels on the iris (rubeosis iridis).

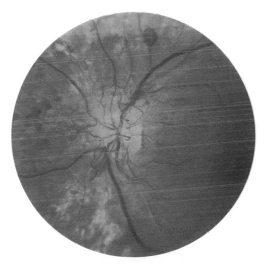

Figure 2.34 Severe disc new vessels. Laser scars from panretinal photocoagulation are also present

Management In some patients vision can be partially restored by a specialized form of intraocular microsurgery called pars plana vitrectomy (Figure 2.36).

Cataract

Diabetes is associated with two types of cataract:

1. Senile cataract which develops at an earlier age and may progress more rapidly in a diabetic than in a non-diabetic patient.
2. True diabetic cataract which is very rare. It is caused by osmotic overhydration of the lens and appears as bilateral white punctate or snowflake opacities. In certain cases the lens may become totally opaque (mature) in a few days.

Ocular motor nerve palsies

Diabetes is a common cause of isolated ocular motor nerve palsy, presumably due to interference with the microvascular blood supply to the nerve. In the vast majority of cases spontaneous recovery occurs within a few months.

- Third nerve palsy – diabetes is an important cause of an isolated pupil-sparing third nerve palsy which may be accompanied by severe

periorbital pain. In some cases it is the first clinical manifestation of diabetes.
- Sixth nerve palsy is also fairly common.
- Fourth nerve palsy may occur.

Pupillary anomalies

Occasionally IDDs develop abnormal pupillary reactions with light–near dissociation secondary to an autonomic neuropathy of the pupil.

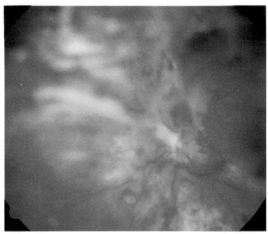

(a)

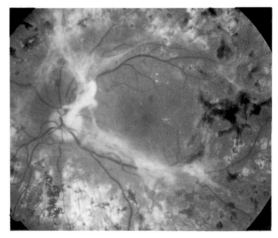

(b)

Figure 2.36 (a) Advanced diabetic eye disease with tractional retinal detachment and vitreous haemorrhage; (b) same eye following pars plana vitrectomy with a flat retina and residual avascular fibrous tissue

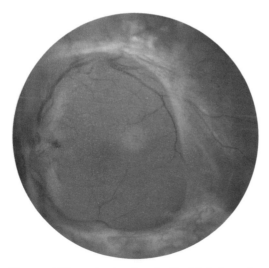

Figure 2.35 Extensive tractional retinal detachment

Changes in refraction

Occasionally unstable diabetics develop fequent changes in refraction. Hyperglycaemia may cause myopia in which the patient suddenly develops blurring of distance vision but is able to read without reading glasses.

Further reading

BLEEKER, G.M. (1988) Changes in the orbital tissues and muscles in dysthyroid ophthalmopathy. *Eye*, **2**, 193–197

BRINCHMANN-HANSEN, O., DAHL-JORGENSEN, K., HANSSEN, K.F. *et al.* (1985) Effects of intensified insulin treatment on various lesions of diabetic retinopathy. *Archives of Ophthalmology*, **100**, 644–653

BRINCHMANN-HANSEN, O., DAHL-JORGENSEN, K., HANSSEN, K.F. *et al.* (1988) The response of diabetic retinopathy to 41 months of multiple insulin injections, insulin pumps, and conventional insulin therapy. *Archives of Ophthalmology*, **106**, 1242–1246

DIABETIC RETINOPATHY STUDY RESEARCH GROUP (1985) Photocoagulation treatment of proliferative diabetic retinopathy. *Ophthalmology*, **88**, 583–600

EARLY TREATMENT DIABETIC RETINOPATHY STUDY RESEARCH GROUP (1985) Photocoagulation for diabetic macular oedema. *Archives of Ophthalmology*, **103**, 1796–1806

FELLS, P. (1987) Orbital decompression for severe dysthyroid eye disease. *British Journal of Ophthalmology*, **71**, 107–111

FELLS, P. (1988) Systemic management of dysthyroid ophthalmopathy. *Eye*, **2**, 198–200

FELLS, P. and McCARRY, B. (1986) Diplopia in thyroid eye disease. *Transactions of the Ophthalmological Society of the United Kingdom*, **105**, 413–423

FINE, S.L. and PATZ, A. (1987) Ten years after the diabetic retinopathy study. *Ophthalmology*, **94**, 739–740

GREY, R.H.B., O'REILLY, N.M. and MORRIS, A. (1986) Ophthalmic survey of a diabetic clinic. I: Ocular findings. *British Journal of Ophthalmology*, **70**, 797–803

HEDIN, A. (1988) Eyelid surgery in dysthyroid ophthalmopathy. *Eye*, **2**, 201–206

JACOBSON, D.H. and GORMAN, C.A. (1984) Endocrine ophthalmopathy: current ideas concerning etiology, pathogenesis and treatment. *Endocrine Review*, **5**, 200–220

JERNELD, B. and ALGVERE, P. (1987) Proteinuria and blood glucose levels in a population with diabetic retinopathy. *American Journal of Ophthalmology*, **104**, 283–289

JERNELD, B. and ALGVERE, P. (1986) Relationship of duration and onset of diabetes to prevalence of diabetic retinopathy. *American Journal of Ophthalmology*, **102**, 431–437

LEONE, C.R. JR (1984) The management of ophthalmic Graves' disease. *Ophthalmology*, **91**, 770–779

MOSS, S.E., KLEIN, R. and KLEIN, B.E.K. (1988) The incidence of visual loss in a diabetic population. *Ophthalmology*, **95**, 1340–1348

NEIGEL, J.M., ROOTMAN, J., BELKIN, R.I. *et al.* (1988) Dysthyroid optic neuropathy. *Ophthalmology*, **95**, 1515–1521

PHELPS, R.L., SAKOL, P., METZGER, B.E. *et al.* (1986) Changes in diabetic retinopathy during pregnancy. Correlations with regulation of hyperglycemia. *Archives of Ophthalmology*, **104**, 1806–1810

SHORR, N. and SIEFF, S.R. (1986) The four stages of surgical rehabilitation of the patient with dysthyroid ophthalmopathy. *Ophthalmology*, **93**, 476–483

WEETMAN, A.P., FELLS, P. and SHINE, B. (1989) T and B cell reactivity to extraocular muscles in Graves' ophthalmopathy. *British Journal of Ophthalmology*, **73**, 323–327

3

Circulatory disorders

Hypertension

Definition

Any definition of hypertension is arbitrary and, to a certain extent, is dependent on the patient's age. In general, the upper limit of 'normal' systolic blood pressure in developed countries is 100 mmHg plus the age of the patient (in some primitive societies there is no substantial increase in blood pressure with age). A diastolic pressure of 100 mmHg or more is considered abnormal in patients less than 60 years of age, and diastolic pressures of 105 mmHg or more are considered abnormal over the age of 60. The two main types of hypertension are: (1) primary (essential) which is the most frequent and has no known cause and (2) secondary which is caused by some other disorder such as renal disease, oral contraceptives, Cushing's disease, phaeochromocytoma, Conn's syndrome, eclampsia and coarctation of the aorta. The 20-year mortality rate in untreated patients with systolic blood pressures over 160 mmHg or diastolic pressures over 100 mmHg is increased by 100% due to (1) stroke, (2) coronary artery disease and (3) congestive heart failure.

Treatment

Antihypertensive therapy is indicated when the blood pressure is consistently above normal limits, particularly if there is evidence of end-organ damage. The aim of treatment is to reduce the blood pressure to within the normal range without producing unacceptable side effects. This is particularly important because treatment is likely to be long term.

General measures

Patients should be encouraged to reduce alcohol intake, stop smoking, lose weight and restrict salt intake. In most patients, however, these measures have only a small impact and drug therapy is required.

Drug therapy

The currently used agents include:

- Diuretics: these should not be used in diabetics and the possible onset of glucose intolerance as a result of these drugs should be checked during therapy.
- Antiadrenergic agents: these should not be used in asthmatics.
- Calcium channel antagonists.
- Angiotensin-blocking agents.

Ocular features

The main ocular complications of hypertension are:

- Hypertensive retinopathy.
- Retinal vein occlusion.
- Retinal artery problems.
- Ocular motor nerve palsy.

Hypertensive retinopathy

The primary response of the retinal arterioles to hypertension is narrowing. However, the degree of narrowing is dependent on the extent of pre-existing replacement fibrosis (involutional sclerosis). For this reason, hypertensive narrowing is seen in its pure form only in young individuals. In older patients the pre-existing involutional sclerosis prevents the same degree of narrowing seen in young individuals. In sustained hypertension the blood–retina barrier is disrupted in small areas resulting in increased vascular permeability. The fundus picture of hypertensive retinopathy is characterized by vasoconstriction, leakage and arteriosclerosis.

Vasoconstriction   The two most important signs are generalized and focal arteriolar narrowing. Unfortunately, the ophthalmoscopic recognition of generalized narrowing may be difficult, but the presence of focal narrowing makes it highly probable that the blood pressure is raised (Figure 3.1). Severe hypertension may lead to obstruction of the precapillary arterioles and the development of cotton-wool spots (Figure 3.2).

Leakage   Abnormal vascular permeability leads to the development of flame-shaped haemorrhages, retinal oedema and hard exudates. The deposition of hard exudates around the fovea in Henle's layer may lead to their radial distribution in the form of a macular star (Figure 3.3) Swelling of the optic disc is the hallmark of malignant hypertension (Figure 3.4).

Arteriosclerosis   Arteriosclerotic features are due to thickening of the vessel wall, which histologically consists of intimal hyalinization, medial hypertrophy and endothelial hyperplasia. The single most important clinical sign is the presence

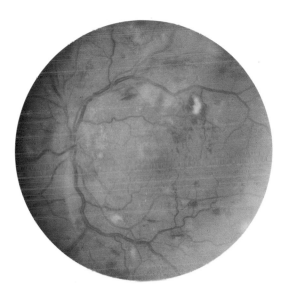

Figure 3.2 Severe hypertensive retinopathy in a diabetic patient with flame-shaped haemorrhages and cotton-wool spots

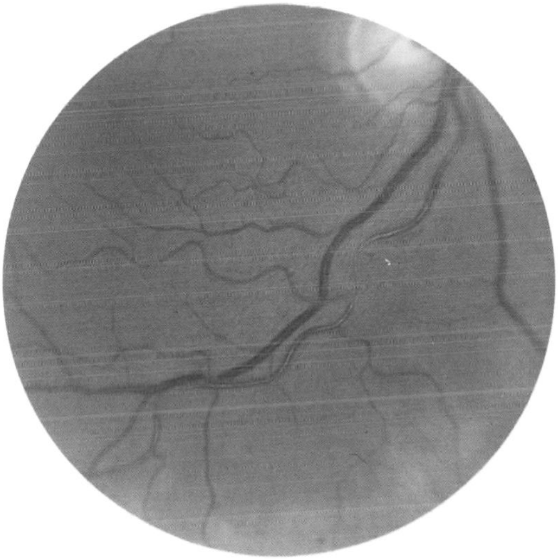

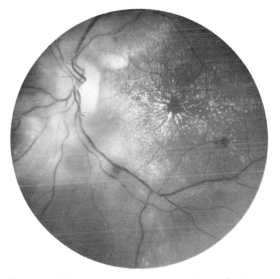

Figure 3.1 Focal arteriolar constriction of the inferotemporal artery due to hypertension (courtesy of Dr N.L. Stokoe)

Figure 3.3 Very severe hypertensive retinopathy in a young person showing generalized arteriolar constriction and hard exudates in the form of a macular star

of marked changes at arteriovenous crossings. Although this feature alone is not necessarily an indication of the severity of hypertension, its presence makes it likely that hypertension has been present for many years. It is also important to point out that mild changes at arteriovenous crossings are seen in patients with involutional sclerosis in the absence of hypertension, and also in normotensive diabetics. The grading of arteriosclerotic features is shown in Figure 3.5.

Grading   The grading of hypertensive retinopathy is as follows:

- *Grade 1*: mild generalized arteriolar constriction. Broadening of the arteriolar light reflex and vein concealment.
- *Grade 2*: more severe generalized as well as focal arteriolar constriction. Deflection of veins at arteriovenous crossings.
- *Grade 3*: flame-shaped haemorrhages, cotton-wool spots and hard exudates. Copper-wiring of arterioles, banking of veins distal to arteriovenous crossings, tapering of veins on either side of the crossings (Gunn's sign) and right-angled deflections of veins.
- *Grade 4*: disc swelling. Silver-wiring of arterioles.

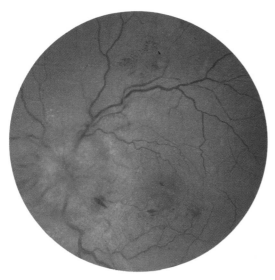

Figure 3.4 Malignant hypertension with marked swelling of the optic disc, a few flame-shaped haemorrhages and severe arteriolar constriction

Retinal vein occlusion

Systemic hypertension is associated with an increased risk of both branch retinal vein occlusion and central retinal vein occlusion. It is postulated that the vein is compressed by the thickened artery where the two share a common adventitia (i.e. at arteriovenous crossings in the retina and just behind the lamina cribrosa in the optic nerve head).

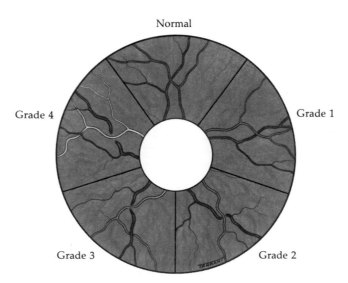

Figure 3.5 Grading of retinal arteriosclerosis

Clinical features

- Acute *branch* retinal vein occlusion is characterized by dilated and tortuous veins, flame-shaped haemorrhages, retinal oedema and cotton-wool spots, affecting the part of the retina drained by the obstructed vein (Figure 3.6).
- In a *central* retinal vein occlusion these changes are more severe and the optic disc may be swollen (Figure 3.7).

Management Although there is no effective treatment for acute retinal vein occlusion, the patient should be referred to an ophthalmologist because some develop secondary neovascularization which requires treatment by laser photocoagulation.

Retinal artery problems

Hypertensive patients may suffer attacks of amaurosis fugax or even retinal artery occlusion as a result of associated arteriosclerosis (see later). Management consists of looking for other associated risk factors such as carotid stenosis, diabetes and hyperlipidaemia

Ocular motor nerve palsies

For details see Chapter 6.

Giant cell arteritis

Definition

Giant cell arteritis is a common, idiopathic vasculitis which typically affects the elderly. The disease has a predilection for large and medium-sized arteries, particularly the superficial temporal, ophthalmic, posterior ciliaries and the proximal part of the vertebral. The severity and extent of involvement is associated with the quantity of elastic tissue in the media and adventitia of the artery. For this reason, the intracerebral arteries, which possess little elastic tissue, are usually spared.

Systemic features

Presentation

This is typically during the seventh and eighth decades of life with the following symptoms:

- Headache is frequently the initial symptom. It develops over a few hours and may be extremely severe and associated with scalp tenderness. The pain may be localized to frontal, occipital or temporal areas, or may be more generalized.
- Blindness is occasionally the presenting feature (see later).

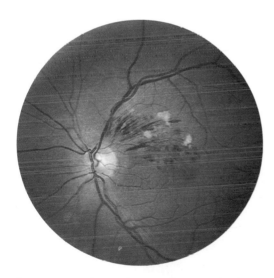

Figure 3.6 Branch retinal vein occlusion with a few flame-shaped haemorrhages and three cotton-wool spots

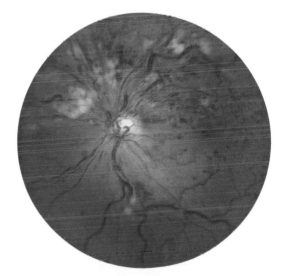

Figure 3.7 Central retinal vein occlusion showing tortuous veins, cotton wool spots and many flame-shaped haemorrhages

- Non-specific systemic symptoms such as weight loss, anorexia, fever, night sweats, malaise and depression are common.
- Jaw claudication due to ischaemia of the masseter muscles which causes pain on speaking and chewing is virtually *pathognomonic*. Occasionally involvement of the lingual artery causes pain in the tongue.
- Polymyalgia rheumatica consists of pain and stiffness in the proximal muscle groups which is worse in the morning and after exertion. Involvement of the shoulder girdle, which makes dressing and combing the hair difficult, is particularly common. Polymyalgia may occur months to years before the cranial symptoms and may not be a prominent feature when headache occurs.

Superficial temporal arteritis

The superficial temporal arteries are tender, inflamed and nodular (Figure 3.8). Initially, pulsation is present although the thickened arteries cannot be flattened against the skull. Later, arterial pulsation ceases and in very severe cases ischaemic gangrene of the scalp may develop (Figure 3.9). The best location to feel for pulsation is directly in front of the upper pole of the pinna of the ear. Lack of pulsation is very suggestive of arteritis because it is most unusual for the superficial temporal arteries to be non-pulsatile in normal elderly individuals. Occasionally, the scalp vessels may appear clinically normal and yet show the typical changes when examined histologically. Although the scalp arteries are classically affected, involvement of other extracranial arteries may also occur.

Miscellaneous uncommon features

- Involvement of the aorta and its main branches gives rise to dissecting aneurysms, aortic incompetence and myocardial infarction.
- Involvement of the vertebral artery may cause brain stem stroke.
- Involvement of the renal arteries may cause renal failure.
- Occult arteritis occurs in some patients in whom systemic features are minimal or absent, and the first manifestations are headaches and unilateral blindness.

Special investigations

Blood

- Erythrocyte sedimentation rate (ESR) is determined largely by elevated fibrinogen levels and the concentration of γ-globins. In giant cell arteritis the ESR is frequently very high, with

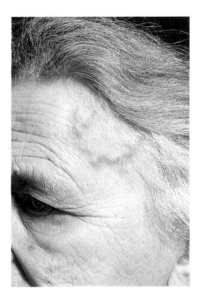

Figure 3.8 Thickened and tortuous superficial temporal artery in giant cell arteritis (courtesy of Dr A. Hall)

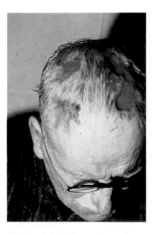

Figure 3.9 Ischaemic scalp necrosis due to giant cell arteritis

levels in excess of 60 mm/h. In interpreting the ESR, it should be emphasized that levels of 40 mm/h may be associated with no apparent abnormality in the elderly and cases of biopsy-proven giant cell arteritis have been reported in patients with ESR levels of less than 30 mm/h. Approximately 20% of patients have a normal ESR.

- C-reactive protein is invariably raised in patients with giant cell arteritis and may be very helpful when the ESR is equivocal.
- Anaemia and an increased white cell count are common.
- Alkaline phosphatase may be elevated.
- Antinuclear antibodies may be present in the serum.

Temporal artery biopsy

Ideally the diagnosis should be confirmed histologically because of the necessity of prolonged steroid therapy (Figure 3.10). Steroids should, however, be started immediately the diagnosis is suspected, and a temporal artery biopsy arranged as soon as possible. Prior treatment with steroids for longer than 7 days may be associated with loss of the histological features of active arteritis. In the presence of ocular involvement it is advisable to take the biopsy from the ipsilateral side. At least 2.5 cm of the artery should be taken, and serial sections must be examined as there may be variations in the extent of arteritic involvement along the length of the artery. Unfortunately,

temporal artery biopsy may fail to confirm the diagnosis in a substantial number of patients. A common difficulty in securing an adequate specimen is the localization of the artery because an inflamed artery frequently loses its pulsation. The ideal location for the incision is the scalp of the temple because this avoids damage to a major branch of the auriculotemporal nerve.

Ocular features

Anterior ischaemic optic neuropathy

By far the most frequent complication which affects about 25% of untreated patients is infarction of the anterior part of the optic nerve, caused by arteritic occlusion of the posterior ciliary arteries. This is referred to as anterior ischaemic optic neuropathy (AION).

Symptoms   Visual loss is typically uniocular, sudden and profound. Its onset may be accompanied by periocular pain, and preceded by visual obscurations and flashing lights lasting a few seconds or minutes. It usually occurs within the first few weeks of the onset of the systemic disease and is extremely rare after the first 9 months have elapsed – hence the need to start steroid treatment as soon as possible. Although simultaneous bilateral involvement is rare, about 65% of untreated patients become blind in both eyes within a few weeks. Once present, visual loss is usually profound and permanent, although very rarely the prompt administration of systemic steroids may be associated with partial recovery. Conversely, in a few unfortunate patients with initially unilateral visual loss, the second eye also becomes blind despite prompt steroid administration.

Signs

- Visual acuity is reduced to hand movements or no light perception.
- Afferent pupillary conduction defect is relative or complete.
- Optic nerve head is swollen, pale and is frequently associated with small splinter-shaped peripapillary haemorrhages (Figure 3.11). Within 1 or 2 months, the swelling gradually resolves and the entire disc becomes pale (Figure 3.12).

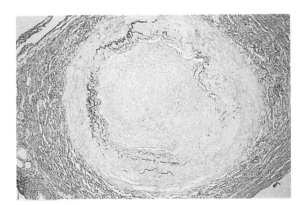

Figure 3.10 Histology of giant cell arteritis: disruption of internal elastic lamina, proliferation of the intima and several giant cells

Differential diagnosis   Other causes of AION:

- Idiopathic type usually occurs in younger patients (45–65 years). It typically causes an altitudinal field defect and the visual loss is less devastating. There is no effective treatment and the second eye frequently becomes involved within several months or years.
- Collagen vascular disorders such as systemic lupus erythematosus and polyarteritis nodosa (see Chapter 5).

Miscellaneous occasional features

- Amaurosis fugax which may be mistaken for that associated with carotid artery disease.
- Central retinal artery occlusion (see Figure 3.17).
- Retinal cotton-wool spots (see Figure 1.13).
- Posterior ischaemic optic neuropathy in which the fundus is initially normal because the ischaemic process is retrobulbar.
- Ocular motor nerve palsies.
- Cortical blindness.

Treatment

The main aim of treatment is to prevent AION in the fellow eye.

- Immediate treatment is with intravenous hydrocortisone 250 mg together with oral enteric-coated prednisone 80 mg. Salt and sugar intakes should be reduced drastically. Prophylactic ranitidine is recommended.
- After 3 days the oral daily dose is reduced to 60 mg for 3 days and then 40 mg for 4 days. The daily dose is then reduced by 5 mg weekly until 10 mg is reached.
- Maintenance daily therapy is 10 mg for 12 months. It is then gradually tapered.
- The duration of treatment is governed by the patient's symptoms and the ESR. Symptoms may, however, recur without a corresponding rise in the ESR and vice versa. The optimal duration for steroid therapy is uncertain. Some patients may only need treatment for 1–2 years whilst others require indefinite maintenance therapy.

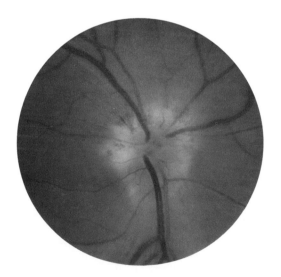

Figure 3.11 Anterior ischaemic optic neuropathy in giant cell arteritis

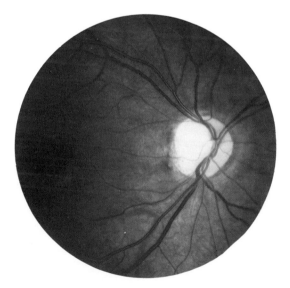

Figure 3.12 Optic atrophy following anterior ischaemic optic neuropathy. Visual acuity is reduced to no light perception

Carotid artery disease

Pathogenesis

Carotid artery disease is a leading cause of morbidity and mortality. The bifurcation of the common carotid artery in the neck into external and internal carotid arteries is an extremely vulnerable site for atheromatous ulceration and stenosis. The irregularity of the vessel wall may be the source of cerebral and retinal emboli composed of *platelets and fibrin* (white emboli) or fragments of atheromatous material including *cholesterol crystals* (Figure 3.13). Severe atheromatous narrowing or occlusion of both carotid arteries may give rise to haemodynamic insufficiency.

Systemic features

Transient cerebral ischaemic attacks

Clinical features A transient cerebral ischaemic attack (TIA) is characterized by a rapid onset of hemianaesthesia, hemiparesis or difficulty with speech lasting less than 24 hours. The majority of TIAs are over within a few minutes. Most cases are caused by thromboembolism from the cervical carotid artery. A haemodynamic cause should be suspected when a TIA coincides with a fall in blood pressure (e.g. on standing up or standing after exercise), especially in patients on hypotensive or antianginal therapy. It should be pointed out that TIAs may also be caused by:

- Thromboembolism from the heart in association with mural thrombi, mitral leaflet prolapse, atrial myxoma, calcific deposits and vegetations (Figure 3.14).
- Vasospasm or temporary vessel wall oedema is thought to be the cause of focal symptoms in migraine and occasionally in hypertension.

Natural history The possible history of untreated TIAs is as follows:

- Spontaneous cessation.
- Persistence of attacks without any residual symptoms, although clinical examination may reveal subtle signs and areas of abnormal signal may be seen on magnetic resonance imaging (MRI).
- Partially recoverable ischaemic neurological deficit (i.e. mild stroke) where clinical features last over 24 hours but resolve within a week.
- Stroke, myocardial infarction or death occurs within 2 years in approximately 15% of patients. A TIA is therefore a dramatic clinical pointer to the state of arteries both focally and generally.

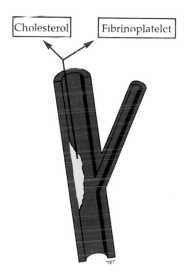

Figure 3.13 Two main types of emboli from carotid artery disease

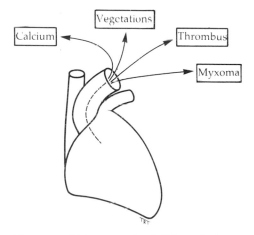

Figure 3.14 Main types of emboli from the heart

Ocular features

Asymptomatic cholesterol crystals

Cholesterol (Hollenhorst's) crystals rarely cause significant obstruction to the retinal arterioles. They appear as minute bright golden to yellow-orange crystals frequently located at arteriolar bifurcations (Figure 3.15). Slight lateral pressure on the globe during ophthalmoscopy may make the presence of unobtrusive crystals clearly visible when the retinal arterioles pulsate.

Retinal transient ischaemic attacks (amaurosis fugax)

Symptoms A retinal TIA is characterized by a painless unilateral loss of vision, often described as a curtain coming down over the eye, usually from top to bottom, but occasionally vice versa. The visual loss, which may be complete, usually lasts a few minutes. Recovery is in the same pattern as the initial loss, although it is usually more gradual. The frequency of attacks may vary from several times a day to one every few months. The attacks may be associated with ipsilateral cerebral TIAs with contralateral signs.

Signs During an attack small grey-white fibrin–platelet emboli may be seen passing rapidly through the retinal arterioles. Associated findings include an afferent pupillary conduction defect and transient retinal oedema. Following an attack of amaurosis fugax the fundus is usually normal, although in some cases cotton-wool spots, or incidental changes such as retinal arteriosclerosis, hypertensive retinopathy or cholesterol crystals, may be seen.

Permanent retinal artery occlusion (retinal stroke)

This may follow a series of amaurosis fugax attacks due to the causes outlined above, or it may occur suddenly without warning. Hypertension is a common finding, with presumed associated atheroma of the central retinal artery or its main branches.

Symptoms These consist of an acute, unilateral, painless and usually permanent loss of vision which is most marked when the central retinal artery is occluded.

Signs

- Impaired visual acuity.
- Relative afferent pupillary conduction defect.
- White, oedematous retina due to ischaemia (Figure 3.16).
- Cherry-red spot at the fovea with central retinal artery occlusion (Figure 3.17a). Later the cherry-red spot disappears and the optic disc becomes pale (Figure 3.17b).
- Arterioles are very narrow and irregular in calibre.
- Blood column in the veins and arterioles is sludgy and segmented (cattle-trucking).

Management of acute retinal artery occlusion
Although the prognosis is very poor the following emergency treatment should be attempted.

- Lie patient flat to help maintain the circulation.
- Apply intermittent firm ocular massage for 15 min to lower the IOP, improve blood flow and dislodge emboli.
- Give intravenous acetazolamide 500 mg to lower the intraocular pressure.
- Other measures include inhalation of a mixture of 5% carbon dioxide and 95% oxygen, and anterior chamber paracentesis.

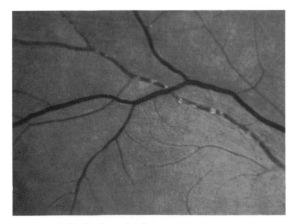

Figure 3.15 Hollenhorst's plaques

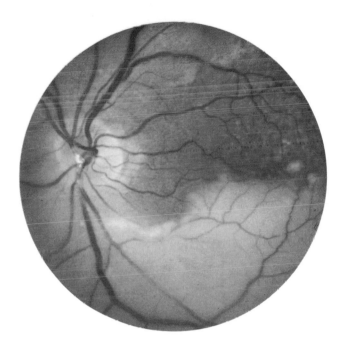

Figure 3.16 Acute inferior branch retinal artery occlusion

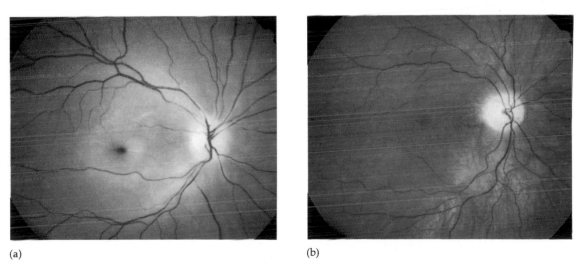

(a)

(b)

Figure 3.17 (a) Acute central retinal artery occlusion with a cherry-red spot at the fovea; (b) same eye 3 months later showing optic atrophy and vascular attenuation

Investigations of carotid disease

All patients should have measurement of blood pressure and urinalysis.

Physical examination

Palpation   The cervical carotid arteries should be gently palpated but not massaged, to avoid dislodging a thrombus. A severe or complete stenosis may be associated with a diminished or absent ipsilateral carotid pulse. Other peripheral pulses may also be abnormal.

Auscultation   A partial stenosis will give rise to a bruit which is best detected with the bell of the stethoscope. It is important to auscultate along the entire length of the artery and ask the patient to stop breathing. The most ominous bruit is one that is high-pitched and soft because it reflects a tight stenosis with a low flow of blood. A loud, low-pitched bruit suggests a large volume of blood flow without much obstruction as in anaemia or thyrotoxicosis. When the lumen is completely obstructed or 90% narrowed, the bruit disappears.

Pressure ophthalmoscopy   The intraocular pressure can be increased by gently pressing on the lateral aspect of the globe during ophthalmoscopy. If the retinal circulation becomes impeded or the central retinal artery is seen to pulsate by relatively gentle pressure, an ipsilateral arterial stenosis is likely. However, negative findings do not exclude a stenosis.

Special investigations

Duplex scanning   This involves a combination of high resolution, real-time, B-scan ultrasonography with Doppler flow analysis. The technique can detect both ulcerative and stenotic lesions and is currently the cheapest available non-invasive test, although it is very operator dependent.

Magnetic resonance imaging   This is likely to become the investigation of choice for visualizing the carotids and demonstrating ischaemic lesions in the brain.

Digital intravenous subtraction angiography   A contrast medium is injected into the superior vena cava via a catheter introduced through the antecubital vein. Images of the carotid arteries are then produced by sophisticated computer-assisted subtraction techniques. The test can be performed on an out-patient basis and is much safer than carotid angiography. Unfortunately the image quality, particularly of the intracranial vessels, is inferior to intra-arterial angiography, but in a cooperative subject with a good cardiac output, satisfactory images of the carotid bifurcation are achieved (Figure 3.18). In only a small proportion of cases is it necessary to proceed to arterial angiography.

Arterial angiography   In most cases, retrograde femoral arteriography is the procedure of choice. Retrograde brachial and direct carotid punctures are less frequently performed. Although arterial angiography (Figure 3.19) is an accurate method of

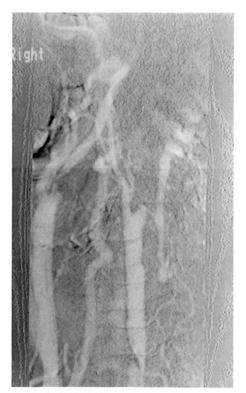

Figure 3.18 Digital intravenous subtraction angiogram showing severe stenosis of the right internal carotid artery and occlusion of the left internal carotid artery (courtesy of Dr J.M. Stevens)

detecting both ulcerative and stenotic lesions, it is associated with a low but significant morbidity. The risk of a vascular event is less than 5% except in individuals suffering from arteriopathy. Using intra arterial digital subtraction techniques, it is possible to use lower volumes of the highly osmotic contrast materials than with conventional angiography.

Management of carotid disease

The aims of management of carotid artery disease are to prevent stroke and permanent visual impairment. The two current modalities are medical therapy and carotid endarterectomy. The chosen method is dependent on the subsequent risk of stroke and also the perioperative morbidity associated with surgical intervention.

Medical therapy

General It is important to emphasize that the presence of occlusive carotid disease is frequently a feature of generalized artherosclerosis. Patients should therefore be screened for associated risk factors such as hypertension, diabetes, hypercholesterolaemia and smoking. Risk factors that are identified should be tackled appropriately. A cardiological assessment may also be advisable.

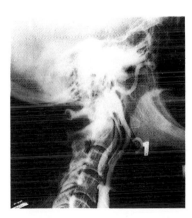

Figure 3.19 Arterial angiogram showing internal carotid artery stenosis (courtesy of Dr J. M. Stevens)

Antiplatelet

- Aspirin reduces the risk of stroke by approximately 20–30%. The optimal dose of aspirin in stroke prophylaxis remains to be defined, but the most frequently used daily dose is 300 mg. Evidence that lower doses than this are effective is awaited.
- Dipyridamole (Persantin) 50 mg three times a day can be used in patients intolerant of aspirin.
- Anticoagulants should be considered if aspirin or dipyridamole fail.
- Fish oils as antiplatelet therapy are yet to be evaluated.

Carotid endarterectomy

In cerebral TIAs The indications for endarterectomy are still controversial. Two large clinical trials are currently in progress on both sides of the Atlantic. Until the results are available, for those clinicians not involved in the trials, the criteria for considering carotid endarterectomy are:

- Failure of medical treatment.
- Inability to take medical treatment (e.g. peptic ulcer).
- Extremely tight carotid artery stenosis (i.e. over 85%).
- Local vascular surgeons' combined morbidity and mortality is less than 3% (since annual stroke rate is 3–8%).

The following factors increase the surgical risk:

- Age over 70 years.
- Coronary artery disease.
- Obstructive pulmonary disease.
- Refractive hypertension.
- Severe obesity.
- Bilateral carotid stenosis and vertebral artery stenosis.

In pure amaurosis fugax Patients with pure retinal symptoms are thought to have a better prognosis than those with hemispherical attacks. The risk of future stroke in untreated patients with isolated amaurosis fugax, cholesterol plaques and retinal infarcts is under 3% per year. These patients should therefore be initially treated with antiplatelet therapy and carotid endarterectomy should be considered only in exceptional circumstances.

Further reading

ADAMS, H.P. JR, PUTMAN, S.F., CORBETT, J.J. *et al.* (1983) Amaurosis fugax: The results of angiography in 59 patients. *Stroke*, **14**, 742–744

ALBERT, D.M., SEARL, S.S. and CRAFT, J.L. (1982) Histologic and ultrastructural characteristics of temporal arteritis: The value of temporal artery biopsy. *Ophthalmology*, **89**, 1111–1126

BECKER, W.L. and BURDE, R.M. (1988) Carotid artery disease. A therapeutic enigma. *Archives of Ophthalmology*, **106**, 34–39

BROWNSTEIN, S., NICOLLE, D.A. and CADERE, F. (1983) Bilateral blindness in temporal arteritis with skip areas. *Archives of Ophthalmology*, **91**, 388–391

BUNT, T.J. (1986) The clinical significance of asymptomatic Hollenhorst plaque. *Journal of Vascular Surgery*, **4**, 559–562

DYKEN, M.L. (1986) Carotid endarterectomy studies: a glimmering of science. *Stroke*, **17**, 355–358

DYKEN, M.L. and POKRAS, R. (1984) The performance of endarterectomy for disease of the extracranial arteries of the head. *Stroke*, **15**, 948–950

GRIFFITHS, R.A., GOOD, W.R., WATSON, N.P. *et al.* (1984) Normal erythrocyte sedimentation rate in the elderly. *British Medical Journal*, **289**, 724–725

HARRISON, M.J.G. and MARSHALL, J. (1982) Prognostic significance of severity of carotid atheroma in early manifestations of cerebrovascular disease. *Stroke*, **13**, 567–569

HEDGES, T.R. III, GIEGER, G.L. and ALBERT, D.M. (1983) The clinical value of negative temporal artery biopsy specimens. *Archives of Ophthalmology*, **101**, 1251–1254

KELTNER, J.L. (1982) Giant-cell arteritis: signs and symptoms. *Ophthalmology*, **89**, 1101–1110

McDONNELL, P.J., MOORE, G.W., MILLER, N.R. *et al.* (1986) Temporal arteritis. A clinicopathologic study. *Ophthalmology*, **93**, 518–530

PATTERSON, R.H. (1988) Stroke. An overview. *Ophthalmology* (Special Article), **95**, 1473–1475

POOLE, C.J.M. and ROSS-RUSSELL, R.W. (1985) Mortality and stroke after amaurosis fugax. *Journal of Neurology, Neurosurgery and Psychiatry*, **48**, 902–903

ROSS RUSSELL, R.W. (Ed.) (1983) *Vascular Disease of the Central Nervous System*. Edinburgh: Churchill Livingstone

ROTH, A.M., MILOW, L. and KELTNER, J.L. (1984) The ultimate diagnosis of patients undergoing temporal artery biopsy. *Archives of Ophthalmology*, **102**, 901–903

TROBE, J.D. (1987) Carotid endarterectomy. Who needs it? *Ophthalmology* (Special Article), **94**, 725–730

WALSH, J., MARKOWITZ, I. and KERSTEIN, M.D. (1986) Carotid endarterectomy for amaurosis fugax. *American Journal of Surgery*, **152**, 172–174

WISNANT, J.P. (1987) Does carotid endarterectomy decrease stroke and death in patients with transient ischaemic attacks? *Annals of Neurology*, **22**, 72–76

4

Rheumatological disorders

Rheumatoid arthritis

Definition

Rheumatoid arthritis (RA) is a very common idiopathic symmetrical and predominantly peripheral chronic inflammatory disorder of the joints. The female to male ratio is 4:1. Eighty-five per cent of patients are positive for IgM rheumatoid factor (seropositive). Seropositive patients have an increased prevalence of HLA-DR4.

Systemic features

Presentation is usually in the fourth and fifth decades of life although rarely the disease can occur in children (juvenile rheumatoid arthritis). The three main ways in which RA presents are:

1. *Insidious onset* over a period of weeks or months – the most common.

2. *Acute onset* over a period of hours or days – occurs in about 10%.

3. *Palindromic rheumatism* – characterized by recurrent attacks of acute arthritis lasting 1 or 2 days.

Arthritis

The arthritis involves the extremities and is usually symmetrical (Figure 4.1). The distal interphalangeal joints are invariably spared as is the axial skeleton with the exception of the cervical spine.

Extra-articular features

● Rheumatoid nodules are the most common extra-articular manifestation of seropositive patients. They consist of firm, round subcutaneous masses most frequently located on the extensor surfaces of the forearms (Figure 4.2).

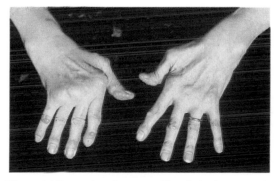

Figure 4.1 Severe involvement of hands in rheumatoid arthritis (courtesy of Dr B. Ansell)

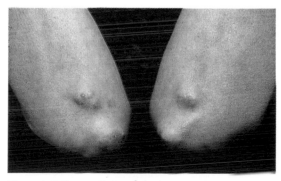

Figure 4.2 Rheumatoid nodules in seropositive rheumatoid arthritis (courtesy of Dr B. Ansell)

- Pleural effusions, interstitial lung fibrosis and nodules (Figure 4.3).
- Felty's syndrome characterized by splenomegaly, thrombocytopenia and leucopenia.
- Acute pericarditis and, rarely, valvular involvement.
- Vasculitis of the skin, peripheral nerves and viscera.
- Secondary amyloidosis may develop in severe long-standing cases.

Treatment

Treatment is mainly with physiotherapy and non-steroidal anti-inflammatory drugs. Disease modifying drugs that are used are anti-malarials, sulphasalazine, gold, D-penicillamine and cytotoxic agents. Systemic steroids are usually reserved for patients with serious extra-articular complications. More than 50% of patients have significant functional disability after 10 years.

Ocular features

Secondary Sjögren's syndrome

Lymphocytic infiltration and secondary fibrosis of the lacrimal glands (Figure 4.4) resulting in a deficiency of tears is by far the most common ocular manifestation, affecting about 20% of patients. The symptoms, signs and treatment are discussed in Chapter 1.

Keratitis

Primary corneal involvement unassociated with scleritis affects about 2% patients. The two main types are:

1. *Peripheral corneal guttering* (contact lens cornea) which is characterized by painless progressive thinning and which may lead to perforation (Figure 4.5).

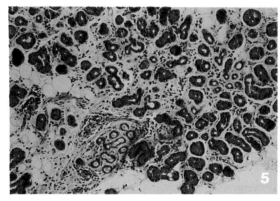

Figure 4.4 Lymphocytic infiltration of lacrimal gland in Sjögren's syndrome

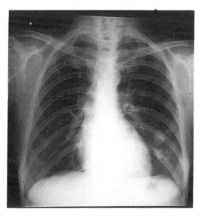

Figure 4.3 Rheumatoid nodules involving the left lower lobe (courtesy of Dr A. Hall)

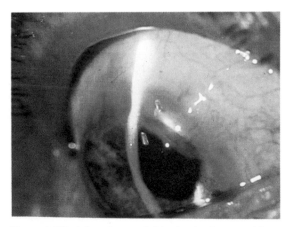

Figure 4.5 Peripheral corneal thinning in rheumatoid arthritis

2. *Keratolysis* which is characterized by acute and severe corneal melting.

Treatment of keratitis is difficult and involves the judicious use of topical steroids and/or systemic steroids and cytotoxic agents.

Scleritis

About 0.5% patients with seropositive RA develop scleritis. The two main types are:

1. *Necrotizing scleritis* with inflammation which is characterized by severe pain, redness and scleral necrosis (Figure 4.6). The adjacent cornea may also be involved. Treatment is very difficult and usually involves systemic steroids or cytotoxic agents.
2. *Scleromalacia perforans* (necrotizing scleritis without inflammation) which is characterized by painless thinning of the sclera leading to exposure of the underlying uveal tissue (Figure 4.7). There is no treatment for this type of scleritis but perforation is uncommon.

Ankylosing spondylitis

Definition

Ankylosing spondylitis (AS) is a common idiopathic chronic inflammatory arthritis that primarily involves the axial skeleton. Symptomatic AS is much more common in males than in females. Patients with AS are negative for IgM rheumatoid factor but are usually positive for HLA-B27 and frequently other family members are affected.

Systemic features

Presentation is typically during the second and third decades with a gradual onset of chronic backache and morning stiffness which is worse on waking and eases with exercise. In some cases acute iritis is the first clinical manifestation of AS.

Arthritis

- Sacroiliitis is usually symmetrical and may be associated with limitation of mobility of the lumbar spine (Figure 4.8).
- Spinal involvement with bony ankylosis is seen in more advanced cases.
- Peripheral arthropathy occurs in 25% of cases and is invariably the presenting feature in children.

Extra-articular features

- Cardiovascular complications are conduction defects and aortitis which may give rise to aortic incompetence.
- Gastrointestinal associations are ulcerative colitis and, less commonly, Crohn's disease.
- Chronic prostatitis is common.
- Apical lung fibrosis is rare but restrictive defects on lung function testing are common because of limitation of thoracic excursion.
- Secondary amyloidosis may occur in severe long-standing cases.

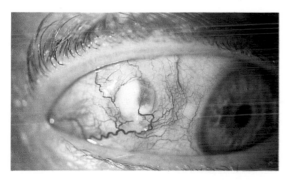

Figure 4.6 Necrotizing scleritis with inflammation in rheumatoid arthritis

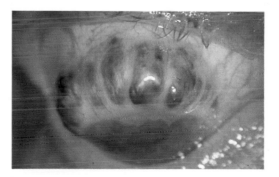

Figure 4.7 Scleromalacia perforans in rheumatoid arthritis (courtesy of Mr B. Mathalone)

Tissue typing

A very strong association exists between HLA-B27, AS and acute iritis. The prevalence of HLA-B27 is as follows:

- In the general population in the UK it is 8%.
- In patients with acute iritis it is about 45%.
- In AS patients it is about 85%.
- In patients with both AS and acute iritis it is about 95%.

Patients with acute iritis, who are HLA-B27 positive but radiologically normal, should be examined by a rheumatologist at 2-yearly intervals because there is a strong likelihood that they will eventually develop AS.

Treatment

Treatment is with physiotherapy and non-steroidal anti-inflammatory agents. In the majority of patients the prognosis is good although a very small minority become seriously physically disabled or have a shortened lifespan due to cardiopulmonary disease.

Ocular features

- Recurrent acute iritis is the typical ocular complication of AS (see Figures 1.6, 1.7, 1.8 and 1.9). Although both eyes are rarely involved simultaneously, either eye is frequently affected at different times.
- The incidence of iritis in patients with AS is about 30% and, conversely, about 30% of males with acute iritis will also have AS.
- There is no correlation between the severity and activity of either eye or joint involvement, and the iritis may either precede or follow the onset of clinical AS. All young adult males with acute iritis should therefore have X-rays of the sacroiliac joints even in the absence of symptoms of AS. This is because in early cases the X-rays may be positive before the patient is symptomatic. The diagnosis of subclinical AS is important because appropriate therapy may prevent the development of severe structural changes in the spine (Figure 4.9).

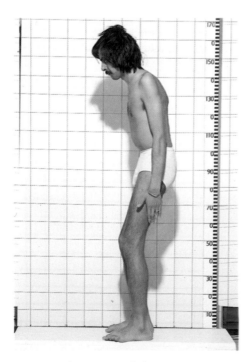

Figure 4.8 Flexion spine deformity in moderately severe ankylosing spondylitis (courtesy of Dr B. Ansell)

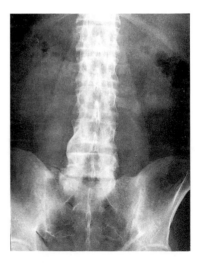

Figure 4.9 X-ray changes in advanced ankylosing spondylitis showing bilateral sclerosis and erosion of the sacroiliac joints, and bony fusion of the spine (courtesy of Dr A. Hall)

Reiter's syndrome

Definition

Reiter's syndrome is a triad of conjunctivitis, urethritis and arthritis. Mucocutaneous lesions are common and spondylitis occurs in some patients. The disease is uncommon and affects males more frequently than females. About 75% of patients are positive for HLA-B27.

Systemic features

Presentation is typically during the third decade with one of the following.

- *Non specific urethritis* - about 2 weeks following sexual intercourse is the most common.
- *Postdysenteric form* which follows an attack of dysentery without a preliminary urethritis.
- *Acute arthritis* may be the first feature in some patients, with either urethritis or dysentery being insignificant.

Arthritis

Arthritis is a major feature of Reiter's syndrome. Most patients recover completely, but in about 15% the arthritis becomes chronic. The arthritis usually affects the lower extremities (i.e. knees and ankles) more frequently than the upper extremities, and the pattern of involvement may be symmetrical or asymmetrical. Some patients subsequently develop sacroiliitis and spondylitis.

Periarticular features

- Plantar fasciitis and Achilles tendonitis are common.
- Bursitis and calcaneal periostitis which may give rise to a calcaneal spur are less common (Figure 4.10).

Extra-articular features

- Painless transient mouth ulcers.
- Scaling plaque-like skin lesions that resemble psoriasis (keratoderma blenorrhagica) have a predilection for the soles of the feet (Figure 4.11).
- Painless erythematous erosion of the glans penis (circinate balanitis) (Figure 4.12)

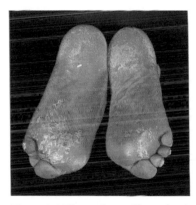

Figure 4.11 Keratoderma blenorrhagica in Reiter's syndrome (courtesy of Dr I. White)

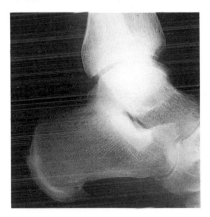

Figure 4.10 Calcaneal spur in Reiter's syndrome (courtesy of Dr A. Hall)

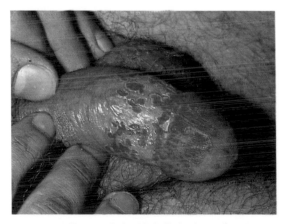

Figure 4.12 Circinate balanitis in Reiter's syndrome

- Non-specific genital ulceration.
- Subungual pustules and thickening.
- Onycholysis with various degrees of thickening and dystrophy (Figure 4.13).
- Nail pitting, which is common in patients with psoriatic arthritis, is uncommon in Reiter's syndrome (see Figure 4.17).
- Cardiovascular lesions include aortitis and first degree heart block.
- Genitourinary lesions include urethritis, prostatitis, cystitis, epidydimitis, orchitis and vaginitis.

Treatment and prognosis are essentially the same as of AS.

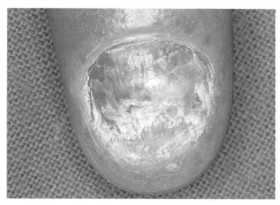

Figure 4.13 Onycholysis in Reiter's syndrome

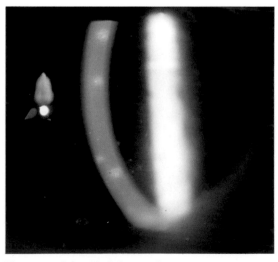

Figure 4.14 Subepithelial corneal opacities in Reiter's syndrome

Ocular features

These are common but usually innocuous.

- Bilateral mucopurulent conjunctivitis is by far the most common ocular manifestation. It usually follows the urethritis by about 2 weeks and precedes the onset of arthritis. The conjunctivitis requires no specific treatment and it usually resolves spontaneously after 7–10 days. Cultures for bacteria are usually negative.
- Acute iritis occurs in about 20% of patients, either with the first attack of Reiter's syndrome or during a recurrence.
- Keratitis may occur in isolation or in association with conjunctivitis. It consists of subepithelial opacities with overlying superficial punctate epithelial lesions (Figure 4.14).

Psoriatic arthritis

Definition

Psoriatic arthritis is an idiopathic, seronegative, chronic, anodular, erosive arthritis that affects about 7% of patients with psoriasis. The disease has no sexual preferential but is associated with an increased prevalence of HLA-B27 and HLA-B17.

Systemic features

Arthritis

Presentation is usually during the fourth and fifth decades with arthritis which is typically asymmetrical and which may give rise to sausage-shaped deformities of the digits (Figure 4.15). A symmet-

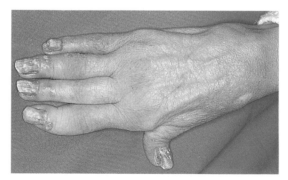

Figure 4.15 Sausage-shaped fingers and severe nail dystrophy in psoriatic arthritis

rical pattern resembling rheumatoid arthritis is, however, occasionally seen and, in some patients, the sacroiliac joints and the spine are also affected.

Extra-articular features

- Psoriasis is usually present before the onset of arthritis (Figure 4.16).
- Nail changes are very common and include pitting (Figure 4.17), transverse depressions and onycholysis.

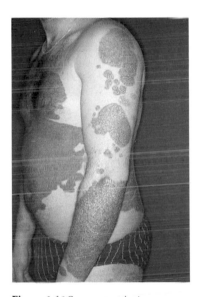

Figure 4.16 Severe psoriasis

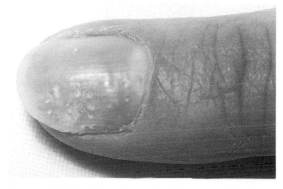

Figure 4.17 Nail pitting in psoriasis (courtesy of Dr I. White)

Treatment

Treatment is with physiotherapy, non-steroidal anti-inflammatory agents and occasionally with gold and D-penicillamine. Cytotoxic agents may also be useful in treating severe skin and joint disease. The prognosis is usually good, although about 5% develop a destructive form of arthritis characteristically involving the distal interphalangeal joints (arthritis mutilans).

Ocular features

- Conjunctivitis occurs in about 20%.
- Acute iritis occurs but is less common than in AS and Reiter's syndrome.
- Secondary Sjögren's syndrome is rare.

Juvenile chronic arthritis
Definition

Juvenile chronic arthritis (JCA) is an uncommon, idiopathic, inflammatory arthritis of at least 3 months' duration developing in children prior to the age of 16 years. The female to male ratio is 3:2. Patients are seronegative for IgM rheumatoid factor. In North America JCA is frequently referred to as juvenile 'rheumatoid' arthritis.

Systemic features

Based on the onset and the extent of joint involvement during the first 3 months the three types of presentation are as follows.

Systemic onset JCA

This accounts for about 20% of cases. In this subgroup the disease is heralded by a high remittent fever and at least one of the following features:

- Transient maculopapular rash (Figure 4.18).
- Lymphadenopathy.
- Hepatosplenomegaly.
- Serositis, predominantly pericarditis.

Initially joint involvement may be absent or mild but the majority of children subsequently develop a polyarthritis. Uveitis is extremely *rare* in this subgroup.

Polyarticular onset JCA

This accounts for about 20% of cases. The arthritis involves five or more joints, most commonly the knees (Figure 4.19), followed by the wrists and ankles. Systemic features are mild or absent and uveitis is *uncommon*.

Pauciarticular onset JCA

This accounts for about 60% of cases. The arthritis involves four or less joints, most commonly the knees, although occasionally only a single finger or toe is affected. Some patients in this subgroup remain pauciarticular whilst others subsequently develop a polyarthritis (i.e. involvement of five or more joints). Systemic features are absent but uveitis is *common* particularly in patients who are positive for antinuclear antibodies.

Treatment

Treatment is mainly with physiotherapy and non-steroidal anti-inflammatory drugs. Occasionally used drugs are steroids, antimalarials, gold, D-penicillamine and sulphasalazine. The prognosis is good and about 75% of patients recover completely by adult life.

Ocular features

Chronic anterior uveitis, which is bilateral in 70% of cases, is the only ocular complication. Because at its onset the uveitis is frequently asymptomatic, it is important to screen those at increased risk at regular intervals so that the uveitis can be treated before it has caused vision-threatening complications (i.e. band keratopathy, cataract and glaucoma – Figure 4.20). Patients with the following

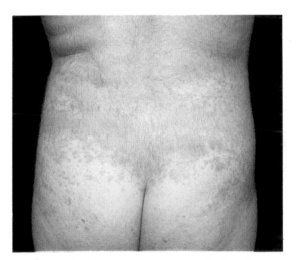

Figure 4.18 Rash in systemic onset juvenile chronic arthritis (courtesy of Dr B. Ansell)

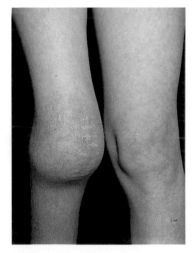

Figure 4.19 Severe involvement of knee in patient with polyarticular onset juvenile chronic arthritis (courtesy of Dr B. Ansell)

features carry an increased risk of eye involvement:

- Pauciarticular onset JCA.
- Girls carry a higher risk than boys by a ratio of 3:1.
- Circulating antinuclear antibodies.
- HLA-DW5 and HLA-DPw2.

Behçet's disease

Definition

Behçet's disease is an uncommon, idiopathic, multisystem disorder which typically affects young men from the eastern Mediterranean region and Japan, but is rare in western Europe and America. The disease is associated with an increased prevalence of HLA-B5. The basic lesion is an obliterative vasculitis probably caused by abnormal circulating immune complexes.

Systemic features

Presentation is usually in the third and fourth decades with recurrent oral aphthous ulceration. Because there are no special confirmatory tests, the diagnosis requires the presence of at least three cardinal lesions, or two cardinal and at least two associated features.

Cardinal lesions

- Oral ulceration is a universal finding and a very common presenting feature. The aphthous ulceration is painful and shallow with a yellowish necrotic base. The ulcers are recurrent and tend to occur in crops. They may involve the tongue (Figure 4.21), gums, lips and buccal mucosa (Figure 4.22).
- Genital ulceration is present in about 90% of patients and is more apparent and troublesome in men than in women (Figure 4.23).
- Skin lesions include erythema nodosum, pustules and ulceration. A papule developing at the site of a skin puncture is characteristic.
- Uveitis (see later).

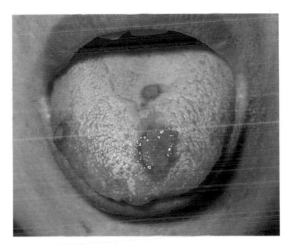

Figure 4.21 Tongue ulceration in Behçet's disease

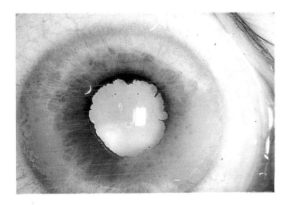

Figure 4.20 Band keratopathy and cataract due to chronic anterior uveitis in pauciarticular onset juvenile chronic arthritis

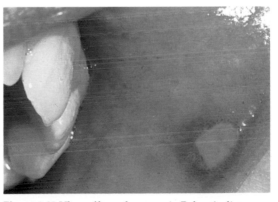

Figure 4.22 Ulcer of buccal mucosa in Behçet's disease

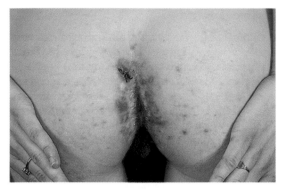

Figure 4.23 Genital ulceration in Behçet's disease (courtesy of Dr I. White)

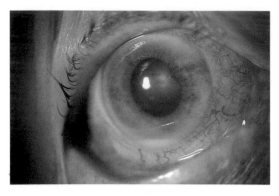

Figure 4.25 Severe anterior uveitis with hypopyon in Behçet's disease

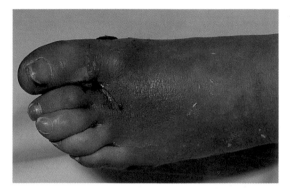

Figure 4.24 Thrombophlebitis in Behçet's disease

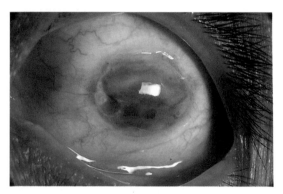

Figure 4.26 Degenerate and blind eye (phthisis bulbi) due to chronic anterior uveitis in Behçet's disease

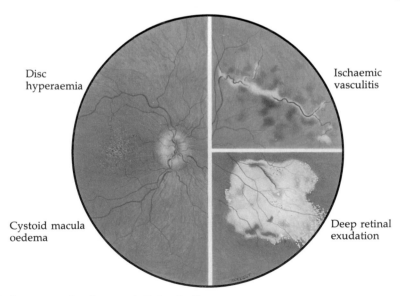

Disc hyperaemia

Ischaemic vasculitis

Cystoid macula oedema

Deep retinal exudation

Figure 4.27 Posterior segment involvement in Behçet's disease

Associated problems

- Thrombophlebitis which may involve the superficial and deep veins including the venae cavae and iliacs (Figure 4.24).
- Arthritis which is asymmetrical, non-destructive and typically affects large joints.
- Gastrointestinal lesions including peptic ulceration and colitis.
- Central nervous system involvement including emotional and mental changes, brain stem syndromes, myelitis, cranial nerve palsies and a low grade meningoencephalitis with organic confusional states.
- Cardiovascular lesions including pericarditis, arterial occlusion, and aneurysms.
- A positive family history for Behçet's disease.

Treatment

Treatment of patients with severe disease is with systemic steroids and immunosuppressants. The prognosis for life in patients with significant CNS involvement is poor. Death may also result from a ruptured aneurysm and pulmonary embolism from deep vein thrombosis.

Ocular features

Ocular complications in Behçet's disease are common and, in patients with involvement of the posterior segment, the long-term visual prognosis is poor.

Anterior uveitis

A non-granulomatous, recurrent, acute, anterior uveitis, which may be associated with a transient hypopyon, is common (Figure 4.25). In many cases the response to topical steroids is good, although in some the uveitis becomes chronic and results in blindness due to phthisis bulbi (Figure 4.26).

Posterior segment involvement

Clinical features (Figure 4.27)

- Diffuse vascular leakage with retinal oedema is the most common and persistent finding.
- Periphlebitis, which may cause venous occlusion and secondary neovascularization, is also frequent.
- Retinitis is in the form of transient white necrotic infiltrates.
- Acute massive retinal exudation associated with obliteration of the overlying blood vessels (Figure 4.28) may lead to areas of retinal necrosis and atrophy (Figure 4.29).

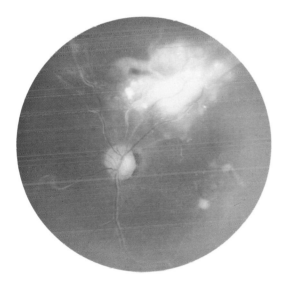

Figure 4.28 Severe retinal infiltration and vasculitis in Behçet's disease

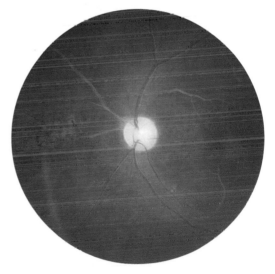

Figure 4.29 Optic atrophy, old vascular sheathing and retinal atrophy in Behçet's disease

Treatment

- The initial treatment is with high doses of systemic steroids which are usually effective in controlling the inflammation. Unfortunately, the lesions subsequently frequently become steroid resistant and require alternative therapy.
- Chlorambucil is initially beneficial in about 75% of cases, but the effects of other drugs such as colchicine and azathioprine are disappointing.
- Cyclosporin A is a potent immunomodulator affecting both the cellular and humoral arms of the immune response. Its use has been shown to be beneficial for the acute exacerbations of both eye and mucocutaneous involvement in Behçet's disease.

Further reading

ANSELL, B.M. (1978) Chronic arthritis in childhood. *Annals of Rheumatic Diseases*, **37**, 107–120

BECKINSALE, A.B., DAVIES, J., GIBSON, J.M. *et al.* (1984) Acute anterior uveitis, ankylosing spondylitis, back pain, and HLA-B27. *British Journal of Ophthalmology*, **68**, 741–745

BENEZRA, D. and COHEN, E. (1986) Treatment and visual prognosis in Behçet's disease. *British Journal of Ophthalmology*, **70**, 589–592

BREWERTON, D.A. (1985) The genetics of acute anterior uveitis. *Transactions of the Ophthalmological Society of the United Kingdom*, **104**, 248–249

COLVARD, D.M., ROBERTSON., D.M. and O'DUFFY, J.D. (1977) The ocular manifestations of Behçet's disease. *Archives of Ophthalmology*, **95**, 1813–1817

GRAHAM, E.M., SANDERS, M.D., JAMES, D.G. *et al.* (1985) Cyclosporin A treatment of posterior uveitis. *Transactions of the Ophthalmological Society of the United Kingdom*, **104**, 146–151

KANSKI, J.J. (1988) Uveitis in juvenile chronic arthritis: incidence, clinical features and prognosis. *Eye*, **2**, 641–645

KANSKI, J.J. (1989) Screening for uveitis in juvenile chronic arthritis. *British Journal of Ophthalmology*, **73**, 225–228

LEE, D.A., BARKER, S.M., SU, W.P.D. *et al.* (1986) The clinical diagnosis of Reiter's syndrome. *Ophthalmology*, **93**, 350–356

MAMO, J.G. (1976) Treatment of Behçet's disease with chlorambucil. *Archives of Ophthalmology*, **94**, 580–583

MICHELSON, J. and CHISARI, F.V. (1982) Behçet's disease. *Survey of Ophthalmology*, **26**, 190–203

MISHIMA, H., MASUDA, K., SHIMADA, S. *et al.* (1985) Plasminogen activator levels in patients with Behçet's disease. *Archives of Ophthalmology*, **103**, 935–936

MOLL, J.M.H., HASLOCK, I., MACREAE, I.F. *et al.* (1974) Association between ankylosing spondylitis, psoriatic arthritis, Reiter's disease, the interstitial arthropathies, and Behçet's disease. *Medicine*, **53**, 343–364

NUSSENBLATT, R.B., PALESTINE, A.G. and CHAN, C.C. (1983) Cyclosporin A therapy in the treatment of intraocular inflammatory disease resistant to systemic corticosteroids and cytotoxic agents. *American Journal of Ophthalmology*, **96**, 275–282

ROSENBERG, A.M. and OEN, K.G. (1986) The relationship between ocular and articular disease in children with juvenile rheumatoid arthritis. *Arthritis and Rheumatism*, **29**, 797–800

WOLF, M.D., LICHTER, P.R. and RAGSDALE, C.G. (1987) Prognostic factors in the uveitis of juvenile rheumatoid arthritis. *Ophthalmology*, **94**, 1242–1248

5

Connective tissue disorders

Systemic lupus erythematosus

Definition

Systemic lupus erythematosus (SLE) is an uncommon, idiopathic, chronic, multisystem, inflammatory disease characterized by striking immunological abnormalities. Organ dysfunction is thought to be caused by circulating autoantibodies and immune complexes. The female to male ratio is 10:1 and the disease is more common in Blacks than in Whites. Patients with SLE have an increased prevalence of HLA-DR2 and HLA-DR3.

Systemic features

Presentation is typically during the third decade with fatigue, weight loss, fever and arthralgia.

Skin

- Butterfly rash consists of facial erythema over the cheeks and nose (Figure 5.1).
- Discoid lesions, consisting of coin-shaped areas of central atrophy and depigmentation with hyperaemic margins, occur in discoid lupus erythematosus which is a related condition that affects only the skin and mucous membranes.
- Miscellaneous and less common findings include bullous and maculopapular eruptions, psoriasis-like lesions, alopecia, digital vasculitis and photosensitivity.
- Raynaud's phenomenon.

Nervous system

Central nervous system involvement occurs in about 50% of patients and includes a variety of neurological and psychiatric features:

- Headache and psychotic reactions are common.
- Seizures, organic brain stem syndrome, strokes, peripheral neuropathy, mononeuritis multiplex and transverse myelitis may also occur.

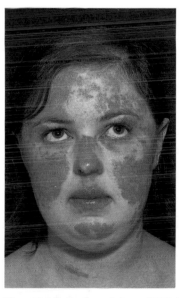

Figure 5.1 Butterfly rash in systemic lupus erythematosus (courtesy of Dr B. Ansell)

51

Kidneys

Renal involvement occurs in 50% of patients and ranges from minimal change nephritis to diffuse proliferative or membranous glomerulonephritis.

Heart

- Pericarditis.
- Myocarditis presenting either with arrhythmias or heart failure.
- Non-bacterial (Libman–Sacks) endocarditis.

Miscellaneous

- Arthralgia and symmetrical arthritis are common. The distal joints are more frequently affected than the proximal, but any joint may be involved.
- Pleurisy, pneumonitis, diffuse interstitial lung disease and the vanishing lung syndrome occur.
- Perforation, infarction and haemorrhage of the bowel may occur as a result of intestinal vasculitis.

Treatment

Treatment of arthritis is with non-steroidal anti-inflammatory agents and antimalarials. The latter are also used for the skin lesions. Patients with severe systemic disease often require systemic steroids. The prognosis for life is very good in the majority of patients.

Ocular features

Anterior segment

- The eyelids may be involved by mucocutaneous disease.
- Punctate epithelial keratopathy unassociated with keratoconjunctivitis sicca is very common.
- Secondary Sjögren's syndrome occurs in about 15% of patients.
- Peripheral corneal thinning is rare.
- Necrotizing scleritis is very rare but it may occasionally be the presenting feature of SLE.

Retinopathy

- Cotton-wool spots, with or without haemorrhages, are the hallmark of SLE retinopathy (see Figure 1.13). Arteriolar dilatation may be present in contrast to cotton-wool spots associated with diabetic or hypertensive retinopathy when arteriolar constriction is the rule. The prevalence of cotton-wool spots appears to correlate with disease activity.
- Occlusion of retinal arterioles is rare. Its pathogenesis is uncertain. It may be due to local disease of the artery wall, embolism or rheological factors producing thrombus in situ. The presence of severe retinal vascular disease is frequently associated with CNS lupus.

Optic (autoimmune) neuropathy

Optic neuropathy affects about 1% of patients. The pathogenesis is probably occlusion of small vessels of the optic nerve. The clinical picture is variable and the condition can present as an acute retrobulbar neuritis, ischaemic optic neuropathy (see Figure 3.11) or slowly progressive visual loss. The possibility of SLE should be considered in virtually all patients, particularly young women, who develop optic neuropathy, as it may be the presenting manifestation. The visual outcome is variable and some cases are responsive to systemic steroids.

Systemic sclerosis

Definition

Systemic sclerosis (scleroderma) is a rare, idiopathic, connective tissue disease characterized by widespread small vessel obliteration and fibrosis of the skin and internal organs. The condition affects females more frequently than males.

Systemic features

Presentation is usually in adult life with Raynaud's phenomenon, distal skin thickening and internal organ involvement.

Skin

The vast majority of patients present with skin involvement. In the early oedematous stages the skin is swollen. Later it becomes tight, waxy, inflexible and adherent to the underlying tissues (Figure 5.2).

Musculoskeletal system

- About 50% of patients have involvement of joints and tendons.
- Myopathy similar to that seen in polymyositis may occur.

Internal organs

- Gastrointestinal tract involvement may affect motility of the oesophagus and small intestine.
- Cardiac involvement may take the form of pericarditis and vasculitis which may cause arrhythmia or heart failure.
- Renal involvement is the leading cause of death.
- Pulmonary involvement may take the form of interstitial lung disease or pulmonary hypertension.

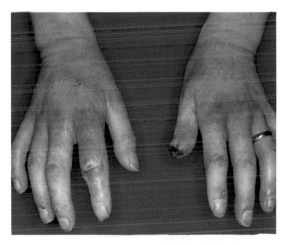

Figure 5.2 Late changes of scleroderma showing tight shiny skin, thinning of the fingers (sclerodactyly), calcinosis of the right proximal interphalangeal joint and a pulp infarction of the left thumb (courtesy of Dr B. Ansell)

Treatment

Treatment is mainly supportive with vasodilators for Raynaud's disease, antacids for oesophageal symptoms, and control of hypertension and heart failure. Although penicillamine is also used, its effects are frequently disappointing and systemic steroids may cause deterioration of renal function. The prognosis for long-term survival is not good.

Ocular features

Ocular manifestations are usually unimportant.

- Eyelid involvement is common and, if severe, it may give rise to problems in blinking and closing the lids.
- Secondary Sjögren's syndrome is uncommon.
- Retinopathy is rare and, if present, it is usually secondary to renal hypertension.

Polymyositis and dermatomyositis
Definition

Polymyositis is an uncommon, idiopathic, inflammatory disease characterized by proximal muscle weakness and tenderness, muscle enzyme elevations, electromyographic changes and inflammatory infiltrates on muscle biopsy. The disease affects females more commonly than males by a ratio of 2:1. When polymyositis is associated with a characteristic skin rash the condition is called dermatomyositis. Children are much more likely to have dermatomyositis than polymyositis. The exact cause is often obscure but the disease is commonly associated with other connective tissue disorders, and it may also result from an underlying malignancy.

Clinical features

Presentation is usually either in childhood or late adulthood with proximal muscle weakness which causes difficulties such as combing the hair and rising from a chair.

Muscles

The characteristic feature is progressive muscle weakness which affects the following muscle groups:

- Proximal muscles of the upper and lower extremities. A late feature in some children with dermatomyositis is contracture of muscles due to the deposition of calcium in the soft tissues around joints.
- Pharyngeal muscle involvement leading to swallowing difficulties.
- Respiratory muscle involvement leading to respiratory failure.
- Cardiac muscle involvement leading to cardiomyopathy.

Skin

Dermatomyositis is characterized by erythematous patches over the face, neck, upper chest and extensor surfaces. Grotton's sign consists of erythematous papules over the metacarpophalangeal or proximal interphalangeal joints (Figure 5.3).

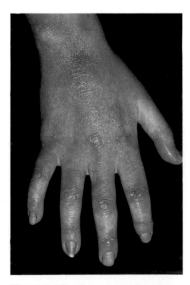

Figure 5.3 Erythematous skin changes in dermatomyositis with collodion patches over the small joints

Miscellaneous

- Interstitial pulmonary disease.
- Arthritis which is mild and symmetrical is uncommon.

Treatment

Treatment is initially with systemic steroids. Cytotoxic agents or plasmapharesis may be helpful in steroid-resistant cases. The prognosis depends on the cause. In adults an underlying malignancy should be sought.

Ocular features

Ocular manifestations are rare and relatively unimportant and are unlikely to be the presenting features of the systemic disease.

- Heliotrope lids are characterized by a violet discolouration. Swelling of the eyelids is common.
- Retinopathy characterized by cotton-wool spots, although rare, is indicative of very severe systemic disease.

Polyarteritis nodosa
Definition

Polyarteritis nodosa (PAN) is a rare idiopathic multisystem disorder characterized by necrotizing arteritis of small and medium-sized blood vessels which leads to thrombosis and aneurysm formation. The male to female ratio is 3:1.

Systemic features

Presentation is usually in the fourth and fifth decades of life with a subacute onset of musculoskeletal or abdominal pain, anorexia, fever, weight loss and skin lesions.

Arteries throughout the body may be involved, leading to widespread changes in many organs.

- Skin ulceration which is slow to heal.
- Arthritis or arthralgia.

- Renal involvement with secondary hypertension – very common.
- Gastrointestinal involvement – may cause mesenteric infarction.
- Lung and heart involvement.
- Peripheral nerve involvement – may cause mononeuritis multiplex.

Treatment

This is with cyclophosphamide and systemic steroids. The prognosis for life is poor with a 50% 5-year survival.

Ocular features

Ocular complications, although uncommon, may be devastating.

Ulcerative keratitis

A bilateral, progressive, necrotizing, peripheral, ulcerative keratitis, although uncommon, may be the presenting feature of PAN. The ulceration usually spreads circumferentially and may also extend centrally. Frequently, it is associated with an adjacent necrotizing scleritis (Figure 5.4) similar to that seen in some patients with rheumatoid arthritis and Wegener's granulomatosis. The keratitis is usually resistant to topical therapy, although systemic treatment of PAN may be beneficial.

Retinopathy

- Occlusion of the central or branch retinal arteries, which may be bilateral, is uncommon (Figure 5.5). Its pathogenesis is uncertain although necrotizing vasculitis is the most likely cause.
- Anterior ischaemic optic neuropathy is rare.

Further reading

DUTTON, J.J., BURDE, R.M. and KLINGELE, T.G. (1982) Autoimmune retrobulbar optic neuritis. *American Journal of Ophthalmology*, **94**, 11–17

GRAHAM, E.M., SPALTON, D.J., BARNARD, R.O. *et al.* (1985) Cerebral and retinal vascular changes in systemic lupus erythematosus. *Ophthalmology*, **92**, 444–448

JABS, D.A., FINE, S.L., HOCHBERG, M.C. *et al.* (1986) Severe vasculo-occlusive disease in systemic lupus erythematosus. *Archives of Ophthalmology*, **104**, 558–563

JAMES, D.G., GRAHAM, E. and HAMBLIN, A. (1985) Immunology of multisystem ocular disease. *Survey of Ophthalmology*, **30**, 155–167

LANGHAM, J.G., BARRIE, T., KOHNER, E.M. *et al.* (1982) SLE retinopathy. *Annals of Rheumatic Diseases*, **41**, 473–478

MORGAN, C.M., FOSTER, C.S., D'AMICO, D.J. *et al.* (1986) Retinal vasculitis in polyarteritis nodosa. *Retina*, **6**, 205–209

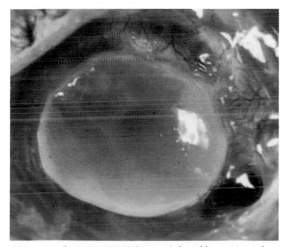

Figure 5.4 Severe necrotizing peripheral keratitis and corneal perforation in polyarteritis nodosa

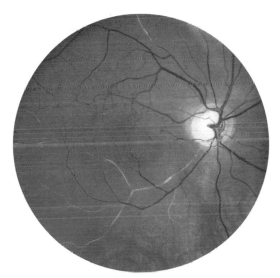

Figure 5.5 Occlusion of retinal arterioles in polyarteritis nodosa

6

Neurological disorders

Myasthenia gravis

Definition

Myasthenia gravis is an uncommon disorder characterized by weakness and fatiguability of voluntary musculature due to impaired transmission at the neuromuscular junction. The female to male ratio is 2:1. The three main types are: (1) progressive, (2) relapsing–remitting and (3) ocular.

Clinical features

Presentation is typically during the third and fourth decades with excessive fatiguability of ocular, bulbar and skeletal muscles. Symptoms are typically worse in the evenings, although some patients may be troubled on first waking.

Ocular features

Ocular involvement is present in 90% of cases and is the presenting feature in 60%.

- Ptosis is bilateral but may be asymmetrical.
- Diplopia is frequently vertical although all or any of the extraocular muscles may be affected.
- Nystagmoid movements may be present on extremes of gaze.
- No pupillary changes.

Non-ocular features

- Bulbar muscle involvement with difficulty in chewing and swallowing.

- Limb muscle weakness which is increased by repetitive movements.
- Involvement of facial muscles may cause a lack of expression.
- Tendon reflexes are normal or exaggerated.
- Absence of sensory changes.
- Permanent myopathic damage may occur in long-standing cases, possibly aggravated by high dose anticholinesterase treatment (pyridostigmine).

Associations

Occasional, associated, acquired autoimmune disorders include: thyroid dysfunction, diabetes mellitus, rheumatoid arthritis, systemic lupus erythematosus, polymyositis, pernicious anaemia, Sjögren's syndrome, pemphigus and sarcoidosis.

Differential diagnosis

Myasthenia is a patchy disease. The differential diagnosis depends on the anatomical site where disease has greatest impact.

Ocular myasthenia

- Ocular myopathy.
- Brain stem demyelination and internuclear ophthalmoplegia.
- Progressive supranuclear palsy.
- Ocular motor palsy.

Bulbar problems

- Guillain–Barré syndrome.
- Motor neurone disease.
- Polymyositis.

Limb weakness

- Guillain–Barré syndrome.
- Myasthenic (Eaton–Lambert) syndrome.
- Polymyositis.
- A myopathy.

Special investigations

Tensilon test

You should *never* do this test on your own. A competent assistant is mandatory and a resuscitation trolley should be close at hand in case of sudden cardiorespiratory arrest (note: Guillain–Barré patients). The test is performed as follows:

- Obtain an objective baseline by measuring the amount of ptosis or the defect in ocular motility defect.
- Inject atropine 0.3 mg intravenously.
- Inject intravenously test dose of 0.2 ml (2 mg) Tensilon (edrophonium hydrochloride).
- Inject the remaining 0.8 ml (8 mg) after 60 seconds provided there is no hypersensitivity.
- Take measurement remembering that the effect of Tensilon lasts only for 5 minutes.

Miscellaneous

- Electromyography may be very helpful in confirming fatigue with repetitive stimulation. This may be combined with the Tensilon injection to clinch the diagnosis.
- Antibodies to antiacetylcholine receptors are present in 90% of cases.
- If antibodies to striated muscle are present the possibility of a thymoma should be considered.
- Chest X-ray of the anterior mediastinum may show a thymic enlargement in 10–20% of patients (usually males).
- CT scan (or preferably MR scan) of the anterior mediastinum should be performed in all patients to rule out the possibility of a thymoma.

Treatment

- Long-acting anticholinesterase drugs (pyridostigmine).
- Systemic steroids.

- Cytotoxic agents (azathioprine, cyclophosphamide).
- Plasmapharesis to remove antibodies in severely affected cases.
- Thymectomy may be helpful in some patients. Young women with generalized symptoms of recent onset are most likely to benefit. Thymectomy should also be performed if a thymoma is suspected.

Myasthenic (Eaton–Lambert) syndrome

Causes

- In association with one of the collagen vascular disorders.
- An underlying malignancy, particularly small cell carcinoma of the lung.

Clinical features

- The weakness may precede other signs of the malignancy by months or even years.
- The limb girdles are characteristically involved, the eye and bulbar muscles rarely.
- Reflexes are typically depressed but enhance dramatically after exercise.
- Repetitive stimulation on EMG produces an increased amplitude of the potentials in sharp contrast to myasthenia gravis.

Treatment

Treatment is of the underlying disorder. Guanethidine hydrochloride may help but anticholinesterases do not.

Ocular myopathies

Definition

These are a group of rare neuropathic or myopathic disorders characterized by slowly progressive ptosis and immobility of the eyes. Some cases are sporadic and others show a dominant inheritance pattern. Muscle biopsy in some patients shows mitochondrial myopathy (inherited through the mother's cytoplasm).

Clinical features

- Bilateral ptosis with a compensatory head tilt (Figure 6.1).
- Chronic progressive external ophthalmoplegia (ocular myopathy), intitially involving upgaze but later all movements may be involved and the eyes virtually fixed. Because muscle involvement is symmetrical diplopia does not occur, even in advanced cases.
- Facial weakness.
- Bulbar involvement with swallowing difficulties occurs in the oculopharyngeal variety.
- Shoulder girdle weakness.
- Kearns–Sayre syndrome in some cases (see Chapter 14).

Dystrophia myotonica
Definition

Dystrophia myotonica is a generalized, dominantly inherited disease characterized by myotonia of skeletal muscles, hypogonadism, frontal balding and presenile cataracts. There is considerable variation in the severity of involvement, even within the same family.

Clinical features

Presentation is usually during the third decade with myotonic features and ptosis. It is also one of the causes of 'the floppy infant'.

Non-ocular signs

- Difficulty in releasing grip. Myotonia is the only common myopathy that affects the peripheral muscles impressively.
- Myopathic facies due to weakness of the facial muscles giving rise to a mournful expression (Figure 6.2). This may be missed because it is easier to overlook a bilateral than a unilateral facial weakness.
- Muscle wasting of the facial muscles, temporalis, masseter, sternomastoid, shoulder girdles, quadriceps and small muscles of the hands.
- Tendon reflexes may be absent.
- Slurred speech due to involvement of the tongue and pharyngeal muscles.
- Hypogonadism with preservation of secondary sexual characteristics.
- Frontal baldness in males.
- Cardiac anomalies.
- Intellectual deterioration.

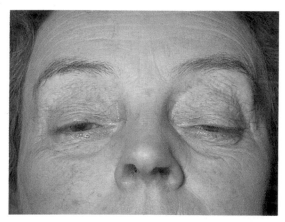

Figure 6.1 Severe symmetrical ptosis in ocular myopathy

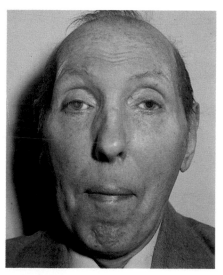

Figure 6.2 Mournful expression of face in dystrophia myotonica. Note right cataract

Ocular signs

- Ptosis which is usually bilateral.
- Presenile cataracts.
- Pigmentary changes at the macula or periphery which are usually innocuous.
- Light–near dissociation of the pupil.

Treatment

- Phenytoin may help the myotonia.
- Surgery for ptosis.
- Cataract extraction and lens implantation.

Multiple sclerosis

Definition

Multiple sclerosis (MS) is a common idiopathic demyelination disorder of the central nervous system characterized by intermittent disturbances of neurological function. It does not affect the peripheral nervous system.

Systemic features

Spinal cord lesions

Common symptoms of MS are weakness, stiffness, muscle spasms, fatigue, sensory disturbances in the limbs, and disturbance of bladder, sexual and bowel function due to plaques of demyelination in the spinal cord.

Brain stem lesions

Plaques of demyelination commonly involve the brain stem and cerebellar connections where they produce diplopia, nystagmus, ataxia, dysarthria and dysphagia.

Hemisphere lesions

Plaques of demyelination in MS tend to occur in the periventricular white matter. MR scanning may show numerous asymptomatic plaques in relatively early clinical cases. Later patients show signs of intellectual decline, depression, euphoria and even dementia. Large plaques may produce sudden hemiparesis, hemianopia and dysphasia.

Transient phenomena

These include epilepsy, Lhermitte's phenomenon (electrical sensation on neck flexion), the transient dysarthria–dysequilibrium–diplopia syndrome, tonic spasms, trigeminal neuralgia, kinesiogenic dyskinesis and Uhthoff's phenomenon (sudden temporary deterioration in symptoms on exposure to heat or after exercise).

Special investigations

Lumbar puncture

The lumbar puncture can be a helpful diagnostic aid in MS. The following findings are suggestive:

- Leucocytosis of 5–50 cells/mm^3.
- IgG level greater than 15% of total protein.
- Oligoclonal bands on CSF protein electrophoresis – commonly in γ4 and γ5 regions. However, this may also be seen in acute infections of the CNS, the Guillain–Barré syndrome and syphilis.

Evoked potentials

Recordings of evoked potentials from the visual, auditory and sensory systems have provided a sensitive way of identifying lesions which may be subclinical. The visually evoked potential is the most frequently used. It involves the stimulation of the retina by a pattern 'checkboard stimulus', and measurement and timing of the electric signal recorded over the visual cortex (Figure 6.3).

CT and MR scanning

- On CT, plaques due to MS show variable enhancement after the injection of contrast medium. The highest yield in detecting plaques is obtained by a double dose of contrast followed by delayed scans. This still visualizes lesions in only about 50% of patients with either probable or definite MS.
- MR is the method of choice because it shows the typical periventricular and brain stem plaques of MS very much better than CT (Figure 6.4). The lesions are seen as bright areas of abnormal signal on T2-weighted and proton density scans. However, in patients with optic neuritis MR may or may not show a plaque within the

Pattern changes

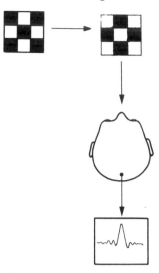

Figure 6.3 Visually evoked potentials. The time taken for the pattern change to register over the visual cortex is measured. The latency is increased in MS

optic nerve (Figure 6.5). Very occasionally patients with clinically probable MS and a positive oligoclonal pattern on CSF electrophoresis will have a negative MR scan of the brain.

Ocular features

Optic neuritis

Prevalence A close association exists between optic neuritis and MS.

- Seventy–four per cent of women and 34% of men with optic neuritis may ultimately develop other neurological dysfunction and be classified as having MS when followed up for 15 years.
- Evidence of optic neuritis may be found in 70% of established MS cases.
- Between 50% and 70% of patients with clinically isolated optic neuritis have abnormal MRI with a distribution of white matter lesions similar to that seen in MS (i.e. periventricular and brain stem).

A strong case can therefore be made for optic neuritis being a forme fruste of MS based on

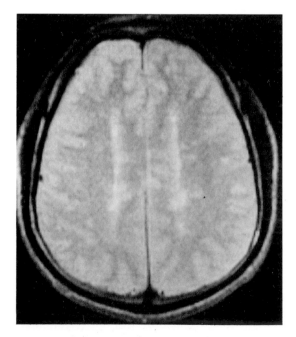

Figure 6.4 MR scan in multiple sclerosis showing white areas of abnormal signal distributed in the deep white matter of both hemispheres, particularly adjacent to the ventricles

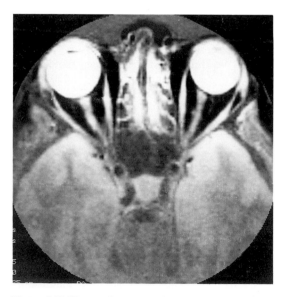

Figure 6.5 MR scan showing a plaque of demyelination in one optic nerve in a patient with retrobulbar neuritis (courtesy of Professor I. McDonald)

similarities between the two conditions in incidence, CSF findings, histocompatibility data, changes present at MR and family history.

Risk of subsequent MS This is increased with:

- Winter onset.
- HLA-DR2 positive.
- Uhthoff's phenomenon in which visual acuity worsens when body temperature rises or during physical exercise.

Note: Optic neuritis may occur with one of the common childhood infections or glandular fever in which case the risk of MS is negligible.

Clinical features

Symptoms A typical attack of optic neuritis starts with an acute onset of monocular visual loss which is frequently associated with periocular discomfort made worse on moving the eye. Visual impairment is progressive and maximal at the end of the second week and often recovers after 4–6 weeks, but it may be slower than this and recovery is sometimes incomplete.

Signs Optic neuritis exerts a filter-like effect on all aspects of visual function as follows:

- Visual acuity is variably impaired.
- Relative afferent pupillary conduction defect is present.

- Colour vision is impaired, even in mild cases.
- Light brightness appreciation is decreased.
- Ophthalmoscopy is normal in the more common retrobulbar form (Figure 6.6). In the less common optic papillitis, the optic disc is swollen (Figure 6.7) and occasionally haemorrhages may be seen.

Treatment Treatment is usually unnecessary although steroids speed up the rate of recovery of vision without affecting the final visual acuity. Intravenous megadose steroids may also alter the course of visual disability from optic neuritis of unknown aetiology. Improvement may be dramatic, particularly in patients with a duration of less than 6 weeks and swollen optic discs. The therapeutic regimens are:

- Oral enteric-coated prednisone (1 mg/kg per day for 14 days).
- Intravenous methylprednisolone sodium succinate (1000 mg/day for 3 days) followed by oral enteric-coated prednisone for 11 days.
- Retrobulbar injection of triamcinolone acetonide 40 mg.

Ocular motility defects

Internuclear ophthalmoplegia All horizontal eye movements are generated from the pontine paramedian reticular formation (PPRF). From here the output is to the *ipsilateral* sixth nerve nucleus

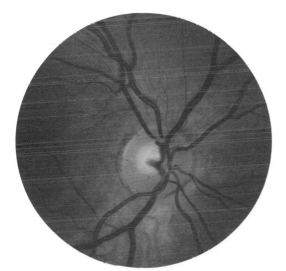

Figure 6.6 Normal optic disc in retrobulbar neuritis

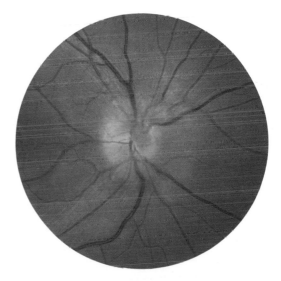

Figure 6.7 Swollen optic disc in optic papillitis

and also to the *contralateral* third nerve nuclear complex via the medial longitudinal bundle (fasciculus) (Figure 6.8). Lesions of the medial longitudinal bundle cause an internuclear ophthalmoplegia which is characterized by:

- Defective adduction of the ipsilateral eye.
- Ataxic nystagmus of the contralateral abducting eye.
- Normal convergence of both eyes when looking at a near object.

Unilateral internuclear ophthalmoplegia may also be caused by brain stem vascular diseases whereas bilateral involvement is usually caused by MS.

Miscellaneous

- Conjugate gaze paresis and skew deviation.
- Isolated ocular motor nerve palsies.
- Nystagmus which is sometimes vertical or rotatory. In some cases the patient is aware of the nystagmus (oscillopsia). This is particularly troublesome when the nystagmus is vertical.

Retinal vasculitis

An occasional finding is a mild asymptomatic retinal vasculitis affecting a segment of one of the peripheral retinal veins (Figure 6.9).

Abnormalities of the pupil

Applied anatomy

Light reflex

The pupillary light reflex consists of *four* neurones (Figure 6.10).

First neurone   This connects the retina with the pretectal nucleus in the midbrain at the level of the superior colliculus. The reflex is mediated by the retinal photoreceptors.

- Impulses originating from the nasal retina are conducted by fibres which decussate in the chiasm and pass up the optic tract to terminate in the *contralateral* pretectal nucleus.
- Impulses originating in the temporal retina are conducted by uncrossed fibres which terminate in the *ipsilateral* pretectal nucleus.

Second neurone   This internuncial neurone connects the pretectal nucleus to *both* Edinger–Westphal nuclei. This is why a unilateral light stimulus evokes a bilateral and symmetrical pupillary constriction. Damage to the internuncial neurones is thought to be responsible for light–near dissociation in neurosyphilis and pinealomas.

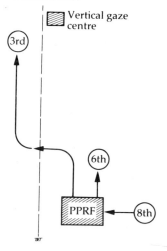

Figure 6.8 Anatomy of the medial longitudinal bundle

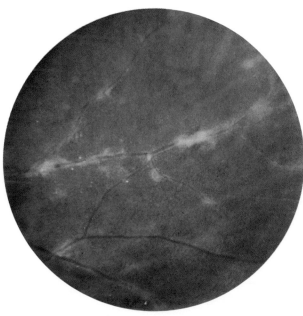

Figure 6.9 Mild peripheral retinal vasculitis in multiple sclerosis

Third neurone This connects the Edinger–Westphal nucleus to the ciliary ganglion. In the orbit the parasympathetic fibres pass in the inferior division of the third nerve, and reach the ciliary ganglion via the nerve to the inferior oblique muscle.

Fourth neurone This leaves the ciliary ganglion and passes with the short ciliary nerves to innervate the sphincter pupillae. The ciliary ganglion is located within the muscle cone, just behind the globe. It should be noted that, although the ciliary ganglion contains other nerve fibres, only the parasympathetic fibres synapse there.

Near reflex

The near reflex triad consists of (1) increased accommodation, (2) convergence of the visual axes, and (3) constriction of the pupils. The term 'light–near dissociation' refers to a condition in which the light reflex is absent or abnormal, but the near response is intact. Vision is not a prerequisite for the near reflex, and there is no clinical condition in which the light reflex is present but the near response is absent.

Anatomical pathway Although the final pathways for the near and light reflexes are the same (i.e. third nerve, ciliary ganglion, short ciliary nerves), the centre for the near reflex is ill defined. There are probably two supranuclear influences: the frontal and occipital lobes. The midbrain centre for the near reflex is probably located in a more ventral location than the light reflex (pretectal nucleus), and this may be one of the reasons why compressive lesions such as pinealomas preferentially involve the dorsal pupillomotor fibres and spare the ventral fibres until late.

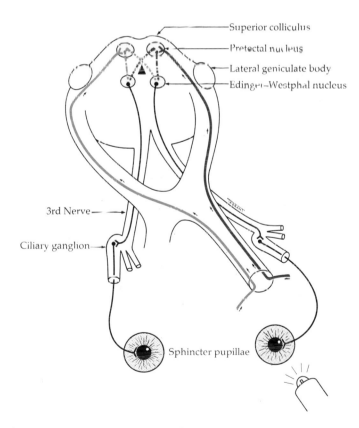

Superior colliculus
Pretectal nucleus
Lateral geniculate body
Edinger–Westphal nucleus
3rd Nerve
Ciliary ganglion
Sphincter pupillae

Figure 6.10 Anatomical pathway of the pupillary light reflex

Sympathetic supply

The sympathetic supply consists of *three* neurones (Figure 6.11).

First neurone This starts in the posterior hypothalamus and descends, uncrossed, down the brain stem to terminate in the ciliospinal centre of Budge (between C8 and T2).

Second neurone This passes from the ciliospinal centre of Budge to the superior cervical ganglion in the neck. During its long course it is closely related to the apical pleura where it may be damaged by bronchial carcinoma (Pancoast's tumour) or during surgery on the neck.

Third neurone This ascends along the internal carotid artery to enter the skull, where it joins the ophthalmic division of the trigeminal nerve. The sympathetic fibres reach the ciliary body and the dilator pupillae muscle via the nasociliary nerve and the long ciliary nerves.

Total afferent pupillary defect (TAPD, amaurotic pupil)

This is caused by a complete optic nerve lesion and is characterized by:

- The eye is completely blind (i.e. no light perception).
- Both pupils being equal.
- Light reflex – when the affected eye is stimulated neither pupil reacts but when the normal eye is stimulated both pupils react normally.
- Near reflex is normal in both eyes

Relative afferent pupillary defect (RAPD, Marcus Gunn pupil)

This is caused by an incomplete optic nerve lesion or severe retinal disease, but not by a dense cataract. The clinical features are those of an amaurotic pupil but more subtle. The difference between the pupillary reactions is enhanced by the *swinging-flashlight test* in which each pupil is stimulated in rapid succession. When the abnormal pupil is stimulated it dilates instead of constricting. This paradoxical reaction of the pupil to light occurs because the dilatation of the pupil, by withdrawing the light from the normal eye, outweights the constriction produced by stimulating the abnormal eye.

Argyll Robertson pupil

This is caused by neurosyphilis and is characterized by the following:

- It is usually bilateral but asymmetrical.
- Pupils are small and irregular.
- Light reflex is absent or very sluggish.
- Near reflex is normal (light–near dissociation).
- Pupils are very difficult to dilate.

Diagnostic difficulties may be encountered in patients with abnormal pupils due to old iritis and diabetics with pseudotabes. Patients with pineal lesions may also have light–near dissociation but the pupils have a normal shape.

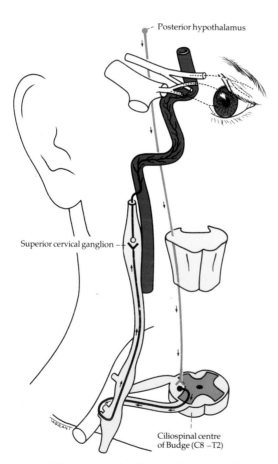

Figure 6.11 Anatomical pathway of the sympathetic nerve supply

Holmes–Adie (tonic) pupil

This is caused by denervation of the postganglionic supply to the sphincter pupillae and the ciliary muscle which may follow a viral illness. The clinical features are:

- It is unilateral in 80%.
- Typically it affects healthy young adults and may be associated with diminished tendon reflexes.
- The affected pupil is large and regular although in long-standing cases it may become constricted.
- Light reflex is absent or very slow.
- Near reflex – constriction is very slow and tonic, and is associated with vermiform movements of the iris; redilatation is also very slow.
- Accommodation is slow.

Pharmacological test

If mecholyl 2.5% or pilocarpine 0.125% is instilled into both eyes the normal pupil will not constrict but the abnormal pupil will constrict (as a result of denervation hypersensitivity). Some diabetic pupils may also show this response and very occasionally both pupils constrict in a normal subject.

Oculosympathetic palsy (Horner's syndrome)

Causes

Disruption of the sympathetic pathways can be by one of the following:

- Pancoast's tumour which may be associated with wasting of the ipsilateral small muscles of the hands, clubbing, tracheal deviation and ipsilateral apical signs.
- Malignant cervical lymph nodes.
- Neck trauma or surgery.
- Brain stem vascular disease or demyelination.
- Carotid and aortic aneurysms.
- Cluster headaches.
- Syringomyelia.
- Idiopathic.
- Congenital.

Clinical features (Figure 6.12)

- Usually unilateral.
- Mild ptosis due to weakness of Müller's muscle.
- Slight elevation of inferior eyelid due to weakness of the inferior tarsal muscle.
- Miosis due to unopposed action of the sphincter pupillae.
- Pupillary reactions are normal to light and near.
- Reduced ipsilateral sweating, but only if the lesion is below the superior cervical ganglion.
- Heterochromia (irides of different colour) is occasionally present if the lesion is congenital.

Pharmacological test

1. Instil *hydroxyamphetamine* 1% (Paredrin) into both eyes:
   (a) in a preganglionic lesion both pupils will dilate;
   (b) in a postganglionic lesion the Horner's pupil will not dilate.
2. Instil *adrenaline* 1:1000 into both eyes:
   (a) in a preganglionic lesion both pupils will not dilate (because adrenaline is rapidly destroyed by amine oxidase);
   (b) in a postganglionic lesion the Horner's pupil will dilate and ptosis may be temporarily relieved (adrenaline is not broken down because amine oxidase is absent).

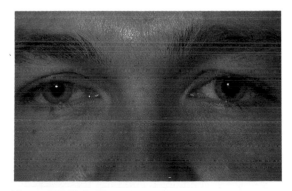

Figure 6.12 Right Horner's syndrome

Nystagmus

Definition

Nystagmus is an involuntary to-and-fro oscillation of the eyes. The three main types are:

1. *Pendular* in which the velocity is equal in each direction.
2. *Jerky* which has a fast and a slow phase. The direction of the nystagmus is designated by the direction of the fast component as follows: right, left, up, down and rotatory.
3. *Mixed* in which there is pendular nystagmus in the primary position and jerky nystagmus on lateral gaze.

Clinical types

Physiological nystagmus

End-point nystagmus   This is a fine jerky nystagmus of moderate frequency found when the eyes are in extreme positions of gaze.

Optokinetic nystagmus   This is a jerky nystagmus induced by moving repetitive visual stimuli across the visual field. The slow phase is a pursuit movement in which the eyes follow the target and the fast phase is a saccadic movement in the opposite direction as the eyes refixate on the target. If the optokinetic tape or drum is moved from right to left, the left parieto-occipital region controls the slow (*pursuit*) phase to the left, and the left frontal lobe controls the rapid (*saccadic*) phase to the right. The optokinetic nystagmus is useful for detecting malingerers who feign blindness and for testing visual acuity in the very young. It may also be helpful in determining the likely cause of an isolated homonymous hemianopia (see Disorders of the optic radiations and visual cortex).

Vestibular nystagmus   This is a jerky nystagmus caused by altered input from the vestibular nuclei to the horizontal gaze centres. The slow phase is initiated by the vestibular nuclei and the fast phase by the brain stem and the frontomesencephalic pathway. Rotatory nystagmus is usually caused by pathological conditions affecting the vestibular system.

Caloric stimulation

- When *cold* water is poured into the right ear the patient will develop a left jerky nystagmus (i.e. fast phase to the left).
- When *hot* water is poured into the right ear the patient will develop a right jerky nystagmus (i.e. fast phase to the right).

A useful mnemonic is 'COWS' (cold–opposite, warm–same).

Motor imbalance nystagmus

This is due to primary defects in the efferent mechanisms.

Congenital

- *Presents* at birth or soon after and persists throughout life.
- *Inheritance* is X-linked recessive or autosomal dominant.
- *Type*: usually jerky and horizontal. It may be dampened by convergence and is not present during sleep. It is usually associated with some impairment of visual acuity.
- It may be associated with abnormal head movements which usually diminish with time.

Spasmus nutans

- *Presents* between the fourth and twelfth month and usually ceases by the age of 3 years.
- *Type*: asymmetrical, pendular, fine, rapid and usually horizontal.
- Associated abnormal head posture and head nodding.

Latent

- *Presents* in early childhood and is common in children with congenital convergent squint (esotropia).
- *Type*: jerky bilateral nystagmus develops when one eye is covered with the fast phase towards the uncovered eye. Occasionally, an element of latent nystagmus is superimposed on a manifest nystagmus so that, when one eye is covered, the amplitude of nystagmus increases.

Ataxic

- *Type*: horizontal jerky nystagmus.
- *Cause*: occurs in the abducting eye of a patient with an internuclear ophthalmoplegia.

Downbeat

- *Type*: fast phase is downwards.
- *Cause*: lesions of craniocervical junction at the foramen magnum.

Upbeat

- *Type*: fast phase is upwards.
- *Causes*: drugs (e.g. phenytoin) and lesions of the posterior fossa.

Convergence–retraction

- *Type*: jerky, in which the fast phase brings the two eyes towards each other in a convergence movement. This is associated with retraction of the globe into the orbit. It is caused by co-contraction of the extraocular muscles, particularly the medial recti.
- *Causes*: lesions of the pretectal area such as pinealomas and vascular accidents. When it is associated with paralysis of vertical gaze, light–near dissociation of the pupils, lid retraction, accommodation spasm, and other midbrain signs, it constitutes Parinaud's syndrome.

See-saw nystagmus of Maddox

- *Type*: one eye rises and intorts whilst the other falls and extorts.
- *Cause*: bitemporal hemianopia usually from a chiasmal lesion.

Periodic alternating

- *Type*: jerky with rhythmic changes in amplitude and direction.
- *Cause*: vascular or demyelinating brain stem lesions.

Sensory deprivation (ocular) nystagmus

- *Type*: horizontal and pendular. Its severity depends on the extent of visual loss and it can often be dampened by convergence. Occasionally an abnormal head posture may be adopted to decrease the amplitude of the nystagmus.
- *Cause*: impairment of central vision in early life (e.g. congenital cataract, macular hypoplasia). In general all children who lose central vision in both eyes before the age of 2 years develop nystagmus.

Third (oculomotor) nerve disease

Applied anatomy

Nucleus

The third nerve nuclear complex is situated in the midbrain at the level of the superior colliculus, inferior to the sylvian aqueduct (Figure 6.13). It is

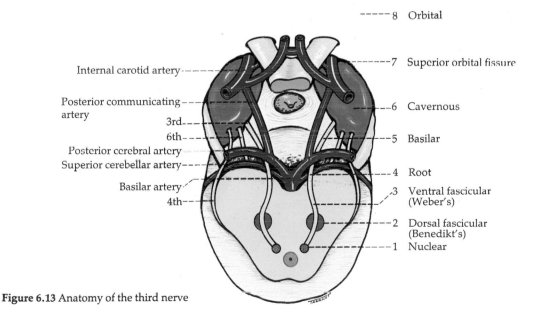

Internal carotid artery

Posterior communicating artery

3rd

6th

Posterior cerebral artery

Superior cerebellar artery

Basilar artery

4th

----- 8 Orbital

------ 7 Superior orbital fissure

-- 6 Cavernous

---- 5 Basilar

---- 4 Root

3 Ventral fascicular (Weber's)

-- 2 Dorsal fascicular (Benedikt's)

-- 1 Nuclear

Figure 6.13 Anatomy of the third nerve

composed of the following paired and unpaired subnuclei.

- The levator subnucleus is an *unpaired* caudal midline structure which innervates *both* levator muscles.
- The superior rectus subnuclei are *paired* and innervate their respective *contralateral* superior rectus muscles. A unilateral third nerve palsy with sparing of the contralateral superior rectus cannot be due to a nuclear lesion.
- The medial rectus, the inferior rectus and the inferior oblique subnuclei are paired and innervate their corresponding *ipsilateral* muscles.

Lesions involving purely the third nerve nuclear complex are relatively uncommon. The most frequent causes are vascular disease, demyelination, primary tumours and metastases.

- Lesions confined to the levator subnucleus cause bilateral ptosis.
- Lesions involving the paired medial rectus subnuclei cause a wall-eyed bilateral internuclear ophthalmoplegia (WEBINO) characterized by defective convergence and adduction.
- Lesions involving the entire nucleus cause an ipsilateral third nerve palsy with ipsilateral sparing of elevation and contralateral weakness of elevation.

Fasciculus

Efferent fibres from the third nerve nucleus pass through the red nucleus and the medial aspect of the cerebral peduncle. They then emerge from the midbrain and pass into the interpeduncular space. The causes of nuclear and fascicular lesions are similar.

- Dorsal fascicular lesion (*Benedikt's syndrome*) involves the fasciculus as it passes through the red nucleus and is characterized by an ipsilateral third nerve palsy and a contralateral hemitremor.
- Ventral fascicular lesion (*Weber's syndrome*) involves the fasciculus as it passes through the cerebral peduncle and is characterized by an ipsilateral third nerve palsy and a contralateral hemiparesis.

Basilar part

The fibres of the third nerve leave the midbrain as a series of 'rootlets' before coalescing to form the main trunk. The nerve passes between the posterior cerebral artery and the superior cerebellar artery. It then runs lateral to and parallel with the posterior communicating artery. Because the nerve traverses the base of the skull along its subarachnoid course, unaccompanied by any other cranial nerve, isolated third nerve palsies are frequently basilar. Important causes are:

- *Aneurysms* at the junction of the posterior communicating artery and the internal carotid artery (Figure 6.14).
- *Extradural haematoma* which may cause a tentorial pressure cone with a downward herniation of the temporal lobe. This compresses the

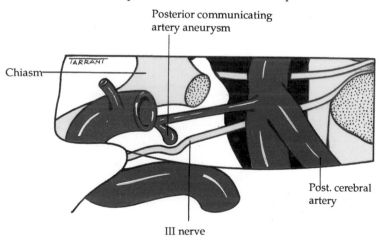

Posterior communicating artery aneurysm

Chiasm

Post. cerebral artery

III nerve

Figure 6.14 Compression of the third nerve by a posterior communicating aneurysm

third nerve as it passes over the tentorial edge (Figure 6.15) and initially causes a fixed dilated pupil followed by a total third nerve palsy.

Intracavernous part

The third nerve enters the cavernous sinus by piercing the dura just lateral to the posterior clinoid process. Within the cavernous sinus, the third nerve runs in the lateral wall and occupies a superior position above the fourth nerve. In the anterior part of the cavernous sinus, the nerve divides into superior and inferior branches which enter the orbit through the superior orbital fissure within the annulus of Zinn. Important causes of intracavernous third nerve palsies are:

- Diabetes.
- Pituitary apoplexy due to haemorrhagic infarction of a pituitary adenoma (e.g. after childbirth) with lateral extension into the cavernous sinus.
- Intracavernous aneurysms and meningiomas.
- Intracavernous granulomatous inflammation (Tolosa–Hunt syndrome) which is characterized by acute or subacute painful ophthalmoplegia.
- Carotid–cavernous fistulae (see later).

Because of its close proximity to other cranial nerves, intracavernous third nerve palsies are usually associated with involvement of the fourth, the sixth and the first division of the trigeminal nerve. The pupil is frequently spared.

Intraorbital part (Figure 6.16)

- The superior division innervates the levator and superior rectus muscles.
- The inferior division innervates the medial rectus, the inferior rectus and the inferior oblique muscles. The inferior branch of the third nerve within the orbit also contains the parasympathetic fibres from the Edinger–Westphal subnucleus, which innervate the sphincter pupillae and the ciliary muscle. Lesions of the inferior division are characterized by limited adduction and depression, and a dilated pupil. The main causes of both superior and inferior division palsies are trauma and vascular disease.

Pupillomotor fibres

The location of the parasympathetic pupillomotor fibres in the trunk of the third nerve is clinically important. Between the brain stem and the cavernous sinus, the pupillary fibres are located superficially in the superior median part of the nerve. They derive their blood supply from the pial blood vessels, whereas the main trunk of the

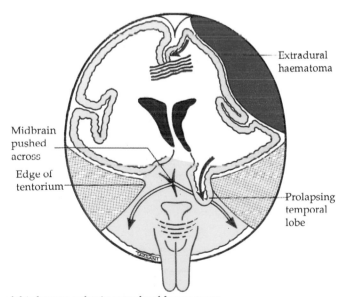

Midbrain pushed across

Edge of tentorium

Extradural haematoma

Prolapsing temporal lobe

Figure 6.15 Mechanism of third nerve palsy in extradural haematoma

third nerve is supplied by the vasa nervorum (Figure 6.17). The presence or absence of pupillary involvement is of great importance because it frequently differentiates a so-called 'surgical' from a 'medical' lesion.

- Pupillary involvement is usually the hallmark of neural compression by *surgical lesions* such as an aneurysm, trauma and uncal herniation, which compress the pial blood vessels and the superficially located pupillary fibres.
- Pupil-sparing third nerve palsies are usually caused by *medical lesions*, such as vascular disease associated with a microangiography which involves the vasa nervorum and causes microvascular neural infarction of the main trunk of the nerve, but spares the superficial pupillary fibres.

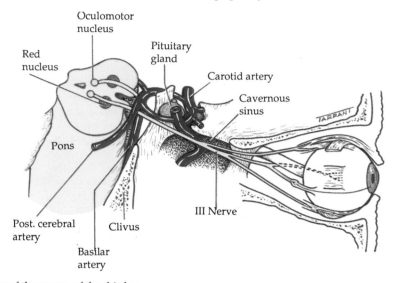

Figure 6.16 Anatomy of the course of the third nerve

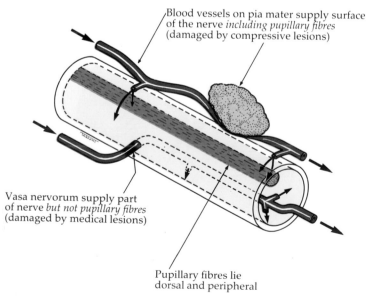

Figure 6.17 Anatomy of pupillomotor fibres within the third nerve trunk

Clinical features of a third nerve palsy

- Weakness of the levator causes ptosis.
- Unopposed action of lateral rectus causes the eye to be abducted.
- Intact superior oblique muscle causes intorsion of the eye on attempted downgaze.

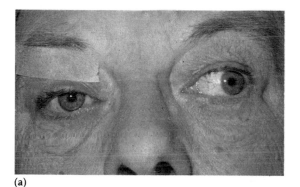

(a)

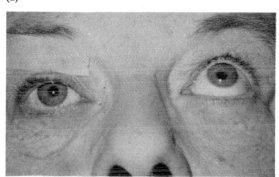

(b)

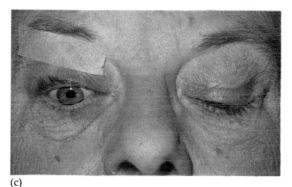

(c)

Figure 6.18 Right third nerve palsy: (a) failure of adduction due to paralysis of the right medial rectus muscle; (b) failure of elevation due to paralysis of the right superior rectus muscle; (c) weakness of depression due to paralysis of the right inferior rectus muscle

- Weakness of medial rectus limits adduction (Figure 6.18a).
- Weakness of superior rectus limits elevation (Figure 6.18b).
- Weakness of inferior rectus limits depression (Figure 6.18c).
- Parasympathetic palsy causes a dilated pupil and defective accommodation (e.g. difficulty in reading small print).

Aberrant regeneration

Secondary aberrant regeneration may occasionally follow acute traumatic and aneurysmal, but not vascular, third nerve palsies. The bizarre defects in ocular motility, such as elevation of the upper eyelid on attempted adduction of depression of the eye, are caused by misdirection of sprouting axons re-innervating the wrong extraocular muscle.

Causes of isolated third nerve palsy

- *Idiopathic* – about 25% have no known cause.
- *Hypertension* and *diabetes* are the most common causes of a pupil-sparing third nerve palsy. In the majority of cases recovery occurs within 3 months. Diabetic third nerve palsies are frequently associated with periorbital pain and are occasionally the presenting feature of diabetes. The presence of pain is not helpful in differentiating between an aneurysmal and a diabetic third nerve palsy because both are frequently accompanied by pain.
- *Trauma* is the second most common cause of a third nerve palsy. However, the development of a third nerve palsy, following relatively trivial head trauma unassociated with loss of consciousness, should alert the clinician to the possibility of an associated basal intracranial tumour which has caused the nerve trunk to be stretched and tethered.
- *Aneurysms* at the junction of the posterior communicating with the internal carotid arteries are a very important cause of an isolated painful third nerve palsy with involvement of the pupil. All patients with these features should be considered for urgent angiography.
- *Tumours, vasculitis* associated with collagen vascular disorders and *syphilis* are uncommon causes.

Special investigations

- *Blood pressure* and *urinalysis* – however, it should be emphasized that the presence of diabetes or hypertension does not exclude the possibility of an aneurysm.
- *ESR* to exclude giant cell arteritis in an elderly patient.
- *Tensilon test* to exclude myasthenia gravis as a cause for a pseudo pupil-sparing third nerve palsy.
- *Forced duction test* to exclude unilateral restrictive thyroid myopathy causing failure of elevation.
- *Arteriography* in an acute painful palsy with involvement of the pupil.
- *CT scanning* in patients with cavernous sinus signs.

Treatment

As with all ocular motor nerve palsies, surgical treatment should be contemplated only after all spontaneous improvement has ceased. This is usually not sooner than 6 months from the date of onset.

Fourth (trochlear) nerve disease

Applied anatomy

- The fourth nerve nucleus is located at the level of the inferior colliculus beneath the sylvian aqueduct (Figure 6.19). It is caudal to, and continuous with, the third nerve nuclear complex. It innervates the *contralateral* superior oblique muscle.
- The axons of the fourth nerve curve around the aqueduct and decussate completely in the anterior medullary velum.
- The nerve leaves the brain stem on the dorsal surface, just caudal to the inferior colliculus. It then curves forward around the brain stem, runs beneath the free edge of the tentorium and (like the third nerve) passes between the posterior cerebral artery and the superior cerebellar artery. It then pierces the dura and enters the cavernous sinus.
- In the cavernous sinus the fourth nerve runs laterally and inferiorly to the third nerve. In the anterior part of the cavernous sinus, it rises and passes through the superior orbital fissure above the annulus of Zinn.
- In the orbit the fourth nerve innervates the superior oblique muscle.

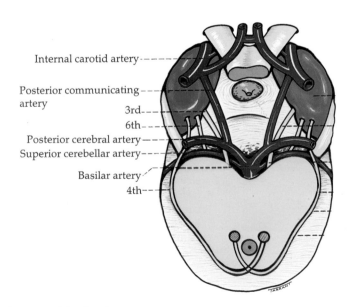

Internal carotid artery

Posterior communicating artery

3rd

6th

Posterior cerebral artery

Superior cerebellar artery

Basilar artery

4th

Figure 6.19 Anatomy of the fourth nerve

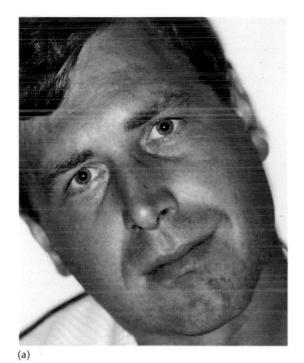

(a)

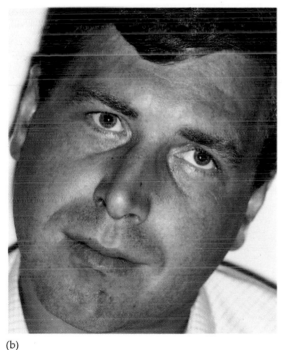

(b)

Figure 6.20 Left fourth nerve palsy: (a) no hyperdeviation on head tilt to the right shoulder; (b) hyperdeviation of the left eye on head tilt to the left shoulder

Important anatomical facts

- The fourth nerve is the longest and slenderest of all cranial nerves.
- It is the only cranial nerve to emerge dorsally from the brain.
- It is the only completely crossed cranial nerve.

Clinical features of fourth nerve palsy

The clinical features of a nuclear, fascicular and a peripheral fourth nerve palsy are clinically indistinguishable and consist of:

- Hyperdeviation (involved eye is higher) due to paralysis of the superior oblique muscle. This is more obvious when the head is tilted to the ipsilateral shoulder (Bielschowsky test) (Figure 6.20).
- Excyclotorsion which is compensatory by a head tilt to the opposite shoulder.
- Limited depression in adduction.
- Diplopia is vertical and worse on looking down. In order to avoid diplopia the patient may adopt an abnormal head posture with a downward head tilt and a face turn to the opposite side.

Causes of isolated fourth nerve palsy

- *Congenital* lesions are frequent although symptoms may not develop until adult life. Examination of old photographs for the presence of an abnormal head posture may be helpful.
- *Trauma* is a very common cause of a frequently bilateral palsy. The nerves may be damaged as they decussate in the anterior medullary velum by impact with the tentorial edge. The nerves can also be damaged as they emerge dorsally and are thrust against the relatively immobile tentorium by contre-coup forces.
- *Vascular* lesions are common but aneurysms and tumours are rare.

Medical investigations are the same as of a pupil-sparing third nerve palsy.

Sixth (abducens) nerve disease

Applied anatomy

Nucleus

The sixth nerve nucleus innervates the ipsilateral lateral rectus muscle. It lies in the midpoint of the pons, inferior to the floor of the fourth ventricle where it is closely related to the fasciculus of the seventh nerve (Figure 6.21). A lesion in and around the sixth nerve nucleus causes:

- Failure of horizontal gaze towards the side of the lesion due to involvement of the horizontal gaze centre in the pontine paramedian reticular formation (PPRF).
- Ipsilateral weakness in abduction due to involvement of the nucleus.
- Ipsilateral facial nerve palsy due to concomitant involvement of the facial fasciculus – also common.

An isolated sixth nerve palsy is never nuclear in origin.

Fasciculus

The emerging fibres pass ventrally to leave the brain stem at the pontomedullary junction, just lateral to the pyramidal prominence.

- Dorsal lesion (*Foville's syndrome*) involves the fasciculus as it passes through the PPRF and is characterized by the following ipsilateral signs: (1) sixth nerve palsy combined with a gaze palsy, (2) facial weakness due to damage to the facial nucleus or fasciculus, (3) facial analgesia from involvement of the sensory portion of the fifth nerve, (4) Horner's syndrome and (5) deafness.
- Ventral lesion (*Millard–Gubler syndrome*) involves the fasciculus as it passes through the pyramidal tract and is characterized by: (1) ipsilateral sixth nerve palsy, (2) contralateral hemiplegia and (3) variable number of signs of a dorsal pontine lesion.

Basilar part

The sixth nerve leaves the midbrain at the pontomedullary junction and enters the prepontine basilar cistern. It then passes upwards close to the base of the pons and is crossed by the anterior inferior cerebellar artery. It then pierces the dura below the posterior clinoids and angles forwards over the tip of the petrous bone, passes through or around the inferior petrosal sinus, through Dorello's canal (under the petroclinoid ligament) to enter the cavernous sinus (Figure 6.22). Important lesions that may damage the basilar portion of the nerve are as follows.

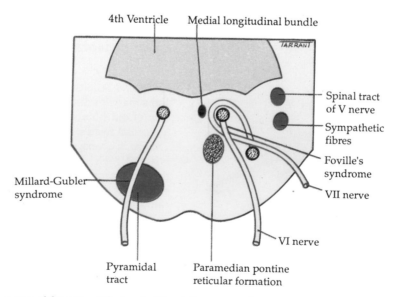

Figure 6.21 Cross-section of the pons at the level of the sixth nerve nucleus

Acoustic neuromas These may damage the sixth nerve as it leaves the midbrain at the pontomedullary junction. It should be emphasized that an early symptom of an acoustic neuroma is hearing loss and an early sign is a diminished corneal sensitivity. It is therefore very important to test hearing and corneal sensation in all patients with sixth nerve palsy.

Nasopharyngeal tumours These may invade the skull and its foramina and damage the nerve during its basilar course.

Chordomas These are rare tumours which arise from notochordal remnants at the clivus. They may cause both unilateral and bilateral sixth nerve palsies.

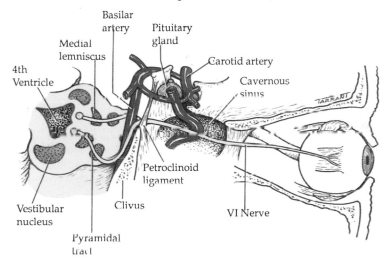

Figure 6.22 Anatomy of the course of the sixth nerve

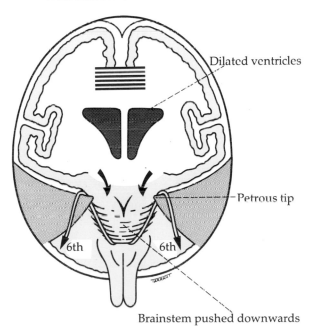

Figure 6.23 Mechanism of sixth nerve palsy in raised intracranial pressure

Raised intracranial pressure This is associated with posterior fossa tumours or benign intracranial hypertension (pseudotumour cerebri) and may cause a a downward displacement of the brain stem. This may stretch the sixth nerve over the petrous tip between its point of emergence from the brain stem and its dural attachment on the clivus (Figure 6.23). In this situation the sixth nerve palsy, which may be bilateral, is a false localizing sign.

Fractures Fractures of the base of the skull may cause both unilateral and bilateral palsies.

Intracavernous part

In the cavernous sinus the sixth nerve runs forwards below the third and fourth nerves. Whereas the latter are protected within the wall of the sinus, the sixth nerve is most medially situated and runs through the middle of the sinus in close relation to the internal carotid artery. It is therefore more prone to damage than the other nerves. Occasionally an intracavernous sixth nerve palsy is accompanied by a postganglionic Horner's syndrome because, in its intracavernous course, the sixth nerve is joined by the sympathetic branches from the paracarotid plexus. The causes of intracavernous sixth nerve and third nerve lesions are similar.

Intraorbital part

The sixth nerve enters the orbit through the superior orbital fissure within the annulus of Zinn to innervate the lateral rectus muscle.

Clinical features of sixth nerve palsy

- Defective abduction due to weakness of the lateral rectus (Figure 6.24a).
- In the primary position there is a convergent strabismus due to the unopposed action of the medial rectus.
- Horizontal diplopia which is worst in the field of action of the paralysed muscle and least away from the field of action of the paralysed muscle (Figure 6.24b).
- Face turn into the field of action of the paralysed muscle in order to minimize diplopia so that the eyes are turned away from this field. For example a patient with a right sixth nerve palsy will turn his face to the right.

Causes of sixth nerve palsy

Most of these have already been described. It should be emphasized that, in contrast to third nerve palsy, aneurysms rarely cause a sixth nerve palsy. Vascular lesions (especially diabetes and hypertension) are, however, common causes.

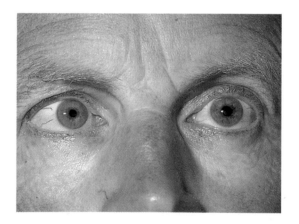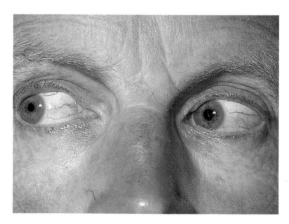

Figure 6.24 Left sixth nerve palsy: (a) failure of left abduction due to paralysis of the left lateral rectus when the patient looks to the left; (b) no deviation on looking to the right

Disorders of the chiasm

Classification

- Tumours:
    Pituitary adenoma.
    Craniopharyngioma.
    Meningioma.
    Glioma.
    Chordoma.
    Dysgerminoma.
    Nasopharyngeal tumours.
    Metastases.
- Non-neoplastic mass lesions:
    Aneurysm.
    Rathke's pouch cyst.
    Fibrous dysplasia
    Sphenoidal sinus mucocele.
    Arachnoid cyst.
    Histiocytosis X.
- Miscellaneous:
    Demyelination.
    Inflammatory.
    Pituitary abscess.
    Trauma.
    Radiation-induced necrosis.
    Vascular.

Applied anatomy

Sella turcica

The pituitary gland lies in a bony cavity of the sphenoid bone called the sella turcica (Figure 6.25). The roof of the sella is formed by a fold of dura mater which stretches from the anterior to the posterior clinoids (diaphragma sellae). The optic nerves and the chiasm lie above the diaphragma sellae and therefore the presence of a visual field defect in a patient with a pituitary tumour indicates suprasellar extension. Tumours confined to the sella will not cause visual field defects. Posteriorly, the chiasm is continuous with the optic tracts and forms the anterior wall of the third ventricle.

Nerve fibres

- The lower nasal fibres traverse the chiasm low and anteriorly. They are therefore most vulnerable to damage from expanding intra-sellar lesions so that the upper temporal quadrants of the visual fields are involved first.
- The upper nasal fibres traverse the chiasm high and posteriorly, and therefore are involved first by lesions coming from above the chiasm (e.g.

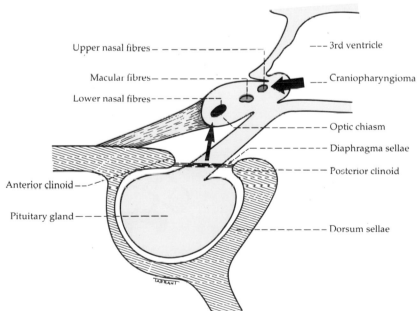

Figure 6.25 Anatomy of the chiasm

craniopharyngiomas). If the lower temporal quadrants of the visual field are affected more than the upper, a pituitary adenoma is unlikely.
- The macular fibres decussate throughout the chiasm.

Variations in location (Figure 6.26)

- In about 80% of normals the chiasm lies directly above the sella so that expanding pituitary tumours will involve the chiasm first.
- In about 10% of normals the chiasm is located more anteriorly over the tuberculum sellae (*prefixed chiasm*) so that pituitary tumours may first involve the optic tracts.
- In 10% of normals the chiasm is located more posteriorly over the dorsum sellae (*postfixed chiasm*) so that pituitary tumours are apt to damage the optic nerves.

Cavernous sinuses

The cavernous sinuses lie lateral to the sella (Figure 6.27a) so that laterally expanding pituitary tumours invade the cavernous sinus and may damage the intracavernous parts of the third, fourth and sixth cranial nerves. Conversely, aneurysms arising from the intracavernous part of the internal carotid artery may erode into the sella and mimic pituitary tumours.

Internal carotid arteries

As the internal carotid artery curves posteriorly and upwards into the cavernous sinus, it lies immediately below the optic nerves. It then ascends vertically alongside the lateral aspect of the chiasm. The pre-communicating portion of the anterior cerebral artery is closely related to the

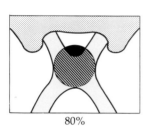 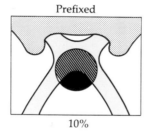 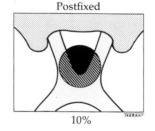

Figure 6.26 Anatomical variations of the normal chiasm

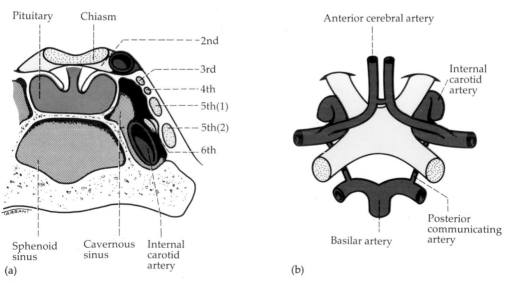

Figure 6.27 (a) Anatomy of cavernous sinus; (b) relations of the circle of Willis with the chiasm

anterior surface of the chiasm and optic nerves (Figure 6.27b). An aneurysm in this region can therefore compress the optic nerve or the chiasm.

Applied physiology of the pituitary gland

The lobules of the anterior part of the pituitary gland are composed of six cell types. Five of these secrete hormones and the sixth (follicular cell) has no known secretory function. The five hormones secreted by the anterior pituitary gland are: (1) growth hormone, (2) prolactin, (3) FSH (follicle-stimulating hormone), (4) ACTH (adrenocortico-trophic hormone) and (5) TSH (thyroid-stimulating hormone).

Hyperpituitarism

Although pituitary adenomas are classified histologically as basophil, acidophil and chromophobe, tumours of mixed-cell types are common and any of the six cell types may proliferate to produce an adenoma (Figure 6.28).

- Basophil tumours secrete ACTH and cause Cushing's disease.
- Acidophil tumours secrete growth hormone which causes acromegaly in adults and gigantism in children.
- Chromophobe adenomas may secrete prolactin and are referred to as prolactinomas. The effect of excessive levels of prolactin in women leads to the infertility–amenorrhoea–galactorrhoea

syndrome, and in men it causes hypogonadism, impotence, sterility, decreased libido, and occasionally gynaecomastia and even galactorrhoea.

- FSH or TSH secreting adenomas are exceedingly rare.
- Some adenomas appear to be non-secreting.

Hypopituitarism

Causes The anterior pituitary is itself under the control of the various inhibiting and releasing factors that are synthesized in the hypothalamus and which pass to the anterior pituitary through the portal system. Pituitary hypofunction may be due to:

- Direct pressure on the secreting cells in the anterior pituitary by a tumour (e.g. an adenoma). Secondary deposits are common in the pituitary but do not normally affect hormonal activity.
- Vascular damage to the pituitary (e.g. pituitary apoplexy after childbirth – *Sheehan's syndrome*).
- Pituitary surgery and/or radiotherapy.
- Interference with the synthesis of inhibiting and releasing factors in the hypothalamus by gliomas.
- Impediment of their transport in the portal system.

Clinical features The clinical picture of hypopituitarism is dictated by the pattern of hormone deficiency and also by the state of growth and development of the patient at the time. Usually gonadotrophin secretion is impaired first, followed by impairment of growth hormone, whilst deficiencies in other hormones occur later.

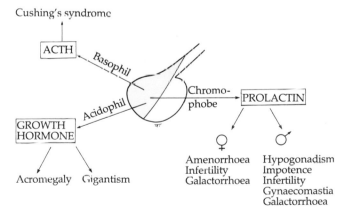

Figure 6.28 Effects of hyperpituitarism

Pituitary adenoma

Clinical features

The chromophobe adenoma is the most common primary intracranial tumour producing neuro-ophthalmological features.

Presentation Pituitary adenomas typically present during early adult life or middle age and only occasionally in the elderly.

- Headache may be the prominent feature due to involvement of pain sensitive fibres in the diaphragma sellae. As the tumour expands upwards and breaks through the diaphragma, the headaches may stop. The nature of the headache is non-specific without the usual features associated with raised intracranial pressure. For this reason delays in diagnosis are common in the absence of obvious endocrine disturbances.
- Bitemporal hemianopic visual field defect usually has a very gradual onset and may not be noticed by the patient until it is well established. It is therefore essential to examine the visual fields in all patients with non-specific headaches or endocrine disturbance.

Visual field defects As the tumour grows upwards it splays the anterior chiasmal notch and compresses the crossing inferonasal fibres causing bilateral superotemporal visual field defects. The defects then progress into the lower temporal fields (Figure 6.29). Because the rate of growth of the tumour is often asymmetrical, the degree of visual field loss is usually different on the two sides. Patients may not present until central vision is beginning to be affected from pressure on the fibres serving the macula. The eye with the greater field loss usually also has more marked impairment of visual acuity.

It should be emphasized that the absence of a visual field defect does not exclude the presence of a pituitary tumour because many remain confined to the pituitary fossa (microadenomas). Acidophil adenomas do not expand beyond the sella as frequently as chromophobe adenomas, and basophil adenomas are usually small and rarely compress the chiasm.

Colour desaturation The earliest sign of a chiasmal field defect is colour desaturation across the vertical midline, which can be detected very simply by using a small red object such as a red pin or a red bottle top (of a Mydriacyl (tropicamide) bottle). The patient is asked to compare the colour and intensity of the target as it is brought from the nasal to the temporal visual field. Another technique is to present simultaneously identical red targets in exactly symmetrical parts of the temporal and nasal visual fields, and to ask if the colours appear the same.

Optic atrophy Optic atrophy is present in only approximately 50% of cases with field defects due to pituitary lesions. Patients are invariably more aware of difficulties with central vision (e.g. when reading) than with peripheral vision, so it is

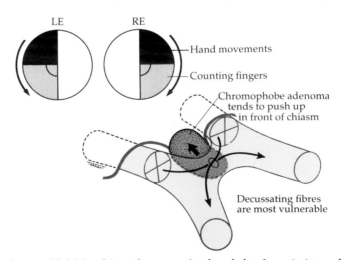

Figure 6.29 Effects on the visual fields by chiasmal compression from below by a pituitary adenoma

extremely important to perform very careful visual field examinations on both eyes in patients with an unexplained unilateral deterioration of central vision.

Miscellaneous

- Diplopia may be due to lateral expansion into the cavernous sinus and involvement of cranial ocular motor nerves. This is particularly likely to occur following pituitary apoplexy.
- See-saw nystagmus of Maddox is a rare finding.

Special investigations

CT scanning (Figure 6.30) This has revolutionized the evaluation of suspected parachiasmal lesions, replacing plain films (Figure 6.31), tomography and pneumoencephalography.

MR (Figure 6.32) This is also very useful in demonstrating the relationship between a mass lesion and the chiasm.

Endocrinological evaluation This should be tailored to the individual patient. All patients suspected of having a pituitary adenoma should have the following evaluated: (1) serum prolactin, (2) FSH, (3) TSH, and (4) growth hormone. An insulin stress test may also be required in selected cases. Patients having large adenomas with visual field defects are at some risk of pituitary apoplexy if the hypoglycaemic response is profound.

Treatment

- The surgical approach to a certain extent depends on the size of the tumour. Small and medium-sized tumours can be approached trans-sphenoidally. Large tumours are best approached transfrontally because this offers the best opportunity to decompress the optic pathways. Very occasionally patients have both a trans sphenoidal hypophysectomy and a craniotomy to remove tissue well above the pituitary fossa.
- Bromocriptine may cause a prolactin-secreting tumour to shrink by causing an increase in secretion in prolactin-inhibiting factor by the hypothalamus. All patients with significant visual field defects should have an urgent prolactin level assay and treatment with bromocriptine should be started as soon as possible. In

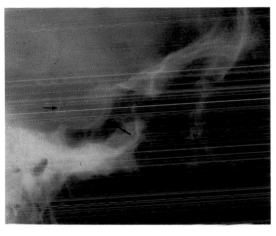

Figure 6.31 Pituitary adenoma causing erosion of dorsum sellae (horizontal arrow) and a double floor to the sella (oblique arrow) (courtesy of Dr I. Yentis)

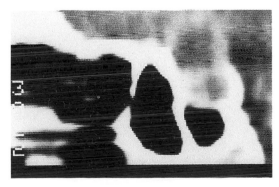

Figure 6.30 CT scan of a prolactinoma with suprasellar extension (courtesy of Dr J.M. Stevens)

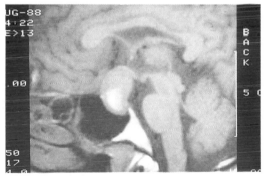

Figure 6.32 MR scan of a large pituitary adenoma with visual field involvement (courtesy of Dr J.M. Stevens)

some patients visual function improves within hours. In many patients endocrine function is also improved with cessation of galactorrhoea, improvement of libido and return of menstruation. It is disappointing that bromocriptine has little useful effect on other pituitary adenomas.

• Radiotherapy may be used alone or in combination with the other two modalities.

Follow-up

As a general rule all patients with chiasmal lesions, irrespective of the cause, should not be discharged from follow-up because in many cases the lesions are often incompletely removed.

• Regular visual field checks and endocrine assessment are necessary.
• Hormone replacement therapy with thyroxine and cortisone is standard after pituitary surgery. Some months after surgery and radiotherapy, a formal endocrine assessment is required to determine if long-term replacement therapy is likely to be required.
• Hydrocortisone supplement at times of intercurrent infection or surgery is required even if long-term hormone replacement therapy is unnecessary.

Craniopharyngioma

Clinical features

Craniopharyngiomas are slow-growing tumours arising from vestigial remnants of Rathke's pouch along the pituitary stalk.

Presentation

• In *children* the tumour may interfere with hypothalamic function and cause dwarfism, delayed sexual development and obesity.
• In *adults* the tumour usually presents with defects in visual acuity and visual fields.

Visual field defects Craniopharyngiomas compress the chiasm from above and behind with initial involvement of the upper nasal fibres, giving rise to bilateral inferotemporal defects. The defects then spread to involve the upper temporal fields (Figure 6.33).

Suprasellar calcification Between 50% and 70% of craniopharyngiomas have suprasellar calcification which can be detected on plain X-rays (Figure 6.34). However, other parachiasmal lesions such as meningiomas, aneurysms and chordomas may also be associated with calcification.

Treatment

Unfortunately, with their local attachments, complete surgical removal is very difficult and recurrences are common. Postoperative radiotherapy may be helpful.

Meningioma

Clinical features

Meningiomas typically affect middle-aged women and frequently cause hyperostosis which can be seen on plain skull X-ray. Visual field defects

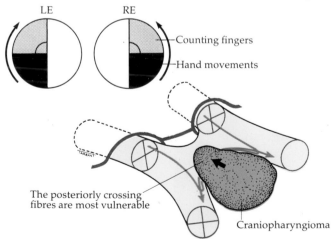

LE   RE

Counting fingers

Hand movements

The posteriorly crossing fibres are most vulnerable

Craniopharyngioma

Figure 6.33 Effects on the visual field by chiasmal compression from above by a craniopharyngioma

depend on the location of the tumour (Figure 6.35).

Tuberculum sellae meningiomas These typically compress the junction of the chiasm with the optic nerve. This gives rise to an ipsilateral central scotoma due to optic nerve compression, and a contralateral upper temporal defect as a result of damage to a loop of contralateral inferonasal fibres which sweeps into the optic nerve before it passes posteriorly (anterior knee of Wilbrand).

Sphenoidal ridge meningiomas These usually cause compression of the optic nerve plus extra-ocular nerve palsies and eventually proptosis.

Olfactory groove meningiomas These may cause loss of the sense of smell as well as compression of the optic nerve.

Treatment

This is surgical, but postoperative radiotherapy is commonly advised in the event of incomplete excision of the tumour.

Miscellaneous chiasmal lesions

Most chiasmal disorders are caused by extrinsic lesions (tumours and aneurysms). However, intrinsic lesions such as glioma, demyelination and trauma may also occur. The chiasm may also be involved by inflammatory or granulomatous lesions such as sarcoidosis, tuberculosis and syphilis.

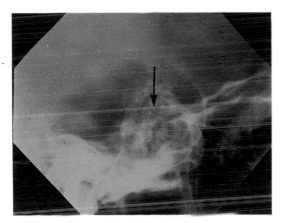

Figure 6.34 Suprasellar calcification in craniopharyngioma (courtesy of Dr I. Yentis)

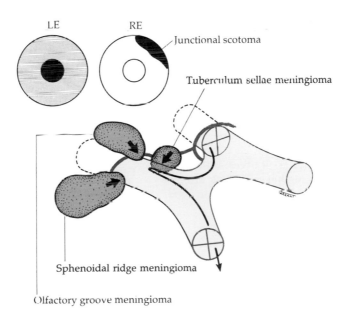

Figure 6.35 Intracranial optic nerve compression by meningiomas and effects on the visual fields by a tuberculum sellae meningioma

Disorders of the optic tract

Applied anatomy

The optic tracts arise at the posterior aspect of the chiasm, diverge and extend posteriorly around the cerebral peduncles, to terminate in the lateral geniculate bodies.

- A lesion that damages the optic tract may also damage the ipsilateral cerebral peduncle and give rise to mild contralateral pyramidal signs.
- Each optic tract contains crossed nasal fibres that originate in the contralateral nasal hemiretina, and uncrossed temporal fibres that originate in the ipsilateral temporal hemiretina. The nerve fibres originating from corresponding retinal elements are, however, not closely aligned. For this reason, homonymous hemianopias caused by optic tract lesions are characteristically incongruous.
- The optic tracts contain both visual and pupillomotor fibres. The visual fibres terminate in the lateral geniculate body, but the pupillary fibres leave the optic tract anterior to the lateral geniculate body, project through the brachium of the superior colliculus to terminate in the pretectal nucleus.
- An optic tract lesion may therefore give rise to an afferent pupillary conduction defect. Characteristically, the pupillary light reflex will be normal when the unaffected hemiretina is stimulated and absent when the involved hemiretina is stimulated. In practice, this *Wernicke's hemianopic pupillary reaction* is difficult to elicit because of scatter of light within the eye, hence the need for a very fine beam of light.
- Because the cell bodies of all fibres in the optic tract are the retinal ganglion cells, optic atrophy may result when the optic tracts are damaged.

Clinical features

- Incongruous homonymous hemianopia.
- Wernicke's hemianopic pupil.
- Optic atrophy.
- Pyramidal signs in some cases.

Causes

Lesions of the optic tracts are relatively rare and are essentially similar to those causing damage to the chiasm (i.e. pituitary adenomas, craniopharyngiomas, meningiomas and aneurysms). The optic tract is particularly vulnerable when the chiasm is prefixed (see Figure 6.26).

Disorders of the optic radiations and visual cortex

Applied anatomy

The optic radiations extend from the lateral geniculate body to the striate calcarine cortex which is located on the medial aspect of the occipital lobe, above and below the calcarine fissure (Figure 6.36). The optic radiations and visual cortex have a dual blood supply from the middle and posterior cerebral arteries, via the carotid and basilar arteries respectively.

- As the optic radiations pass posteriorly, fibres from corresponding retinal elements lie progressively closer together. For this reason, incomplete hemianopias caused by posterior radiations are more congruous than those involving the anterior radiations. However, a complete hemianopia has no localizing value because the extent of congruity cannot be assessed.
- Because the visual fibres synapse in the lateral geniculate body, lesions of the optic radiations do not produce optic atrophy.

Temporal radiation

- The inferior fibres of the optic radiations, which subserve the upper visual fields, first sweep anteroinferiorly in *Meyer's loop* around the anterior tip of the temporal horn of the lateral ventricle, and into the temporal lobe. Lesions in this region classically give rise to an upper quadrantanopia, the so-called 'pie in the sky' defect.
- Because the inferior fibres are very close to the sensory and motor fibres of the internal capsule, a lesion in this area, which is usually

vascular, may give rise to an associated contra-lateral hemisensory disturbance and mild hemiparesis. The inferior fibres then pass posteriorly and rejoin the superior fibres.

Anterior parietal radiation

The superior fibres of the radiations, which subserve the inferior visual fields, proceed directly posteriorly through the parietal lobe to the occipital cortex. A lesion involving only the anterior parietal part of the radiations, which is very rare, will therefore cause an inferior quadrantanopia ('pie on the floor'). In general, hemianopias due to parietal lobe lesions tend to be relatively congruous and either complete or denser inferiorly.

Main radiation

Deep in the parietal lobe, the optic radiations lie just external to the trigone and the occipital horn of the lateral ventricle. Lesions in this area usually cause a complete homonymous hemianopia.

Striate calcarine cortex

- In the striate calcarine cortex, the peripheral visual fields are represented anteriorly. This part of the occipital lobe is supplied by a branch of the posterior cerebral artery.
- Central macular vision is represented posteriorly, at the tip of the calcarine cortex which is supplied mainly by a branch of the middle cerebral artery. Occlusion of the posterior cerebral artery will therefore tend to produce a macula-sparing congruous homonymous hemianopia. Damage to the tip of the occipital cortex, as could occur from a head injury, tends to give rise to congruous homonymous macular defects although asymmetrical macula sparing may sometimes occur with vascular lesions of the occipital lobe.

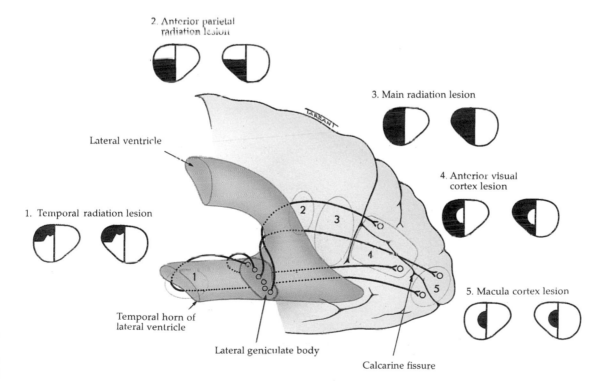

Figure 6.36 Visual field defects caused by lesions of the optic radiations and visual cortex

Associated neurological defects

Temporal lobe

Apart from hemianopias, other features of temporal lobe disease include:

- Paroxysmal olfactory and gustatory hallucinations (uncinate fits).
- Seizures.
- Formed visual hallucinations. These are less likely to be due to schizophrenia where auditory hallucinations are more common.
- Receptive dysphasia.

Parietal lobe

Patients with parietal lobe disease may have:

- Agnosias: visual, colour or sensory (astereognosis).
- Visual perception difficulties, particularly with right parietal lesions.
- Right–left confusion and acalculia, particularly with left parietal lesions.

Visual cortex

Lesions of the visual cortex may cause:

- Formed visual hallucinations, particularly in the hemianopic field. These are thought to be akin to sensory deprivation phenomena and not epileptic.
- Denial of blindness in patients with complete cortical blindness (*Anton's syndrome*). These patients may be reluctant to accept advice not to drive!

Aetiology

Vascular lesions in the territory of the posterior cerebral artery are responsible for over 90% of isolated homonymous hemianopias without other neurological deficits. Other less common causes are migraine, trauma, and primary and secondary tumours.

Optokinetic nystagmus

Optokinetic nystagmus (OKN) may be useful in determining the cause of an isolated homonymous hemianopia that does not conform to any set pattern in patients without associated neurological deficits. If the optomotor pathways in the posterior hemisphere are damaged, the OKN response will be diminished when targets are rotated towards the side of the lesion (i.e. away from the hemianopia). This is called the positive OKN sign.

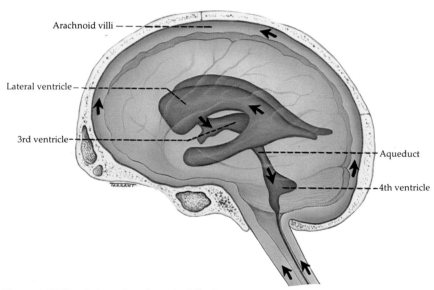

Figure 6.37 Circulation of cerebrospinal fluid

In most cases, the combination of a homonymous hemianopia and OKN asymmetry suggests a parietal lobe lesion, often a neoplasm. Rarely occipital lobe lesions may also cause OKN asymmetry.

Raised intracranial pressure

Circulation of cerebrospinal fluid

- The cerebrospinal fluid (CSF) is formed by the choroid plexus in both lateral ventricles and in the third ventricle (Figure 6.37).
- CSF leaves the lateral ventricles to enter the third ventricle through the foramen of Monro.
- From the third ventricle the CSF flows through the sylvian aqueduct to the fourth ventricle.
- From the fourth ventricle the CSF passes through the foramina of Luschka and Magendie, some flowing around the spinal cord and the rest bathing the cerebral hemispheres.
- Absorption is into the cerebral venous drainage system through the arachnoid villi.

Causes of raised intracranial pressure

- Space-occupying lesions including intracranial haemorrhage.
- Blockage of ventricular system by congenital or acquired lesions.
- Obstruction of CSF absorption via arachnoid villi, previously damaged by meningitis, subarachnoid haemorrhage or cerebral trauma.
- Benign intracranial hypertension (pseudotumour cerebri).
- Severe hypertension.
- Hypersecretion of CSF by choroid plexus tumour (rare).

Systemic features

Headache

This is typically worse in the morning. It tends to get progressively worse and patients usually present to hospital within 6 weeks. The headache may be generalized or localized, and it may intensify with a Valsalva manoeuvre, head movement or bending. Patients with lifelong headaches often report a change in character of the headache. Very rarely will patients have raised intracranial pressure without headache.

Sudden nausea and projectile vomiting

These may be precipitated by fluctuations in intracranial pressure and movement.

Neurological symptoms and signs

These may accompany the headache.

Horizontal diplopia

This is due to stretching of the sixth nerve over the petrous tip (see Figure 6.23).

Papilloedema

Definition

Papilloedema is defined as swelling of the optic nerve head secondary to raised intracranial pressure. It is nearly always bilateral, although it may be asymmetrical. All other causes of disc oedema not associated with raised intracranial pressure (e.g. optic papillitis, central retinal vein occlusion) are referred to as 'disc swelling' and produce an impairment of vision.

Association with brain tumours

All patients with papilloedema should be suspected of having an intracranial mass until the contrary is proved. However, not all patients with raised intracranial pressure will necessarily develop papilloedema, sometimes as a result of an anatomical quirk. Tumours of the cerebral hemispheres tend to produce papilloedema later than those in the posterior fossa. Patients, who have had papilloedema before, may develop a substantial increase in intracranial pressure but fail to re-develop papilloedema because of glial scarring of the optic nerve head. Conversely, not all patients with papilloedema will have a tumour, as some may have benign intracranial hypertension or some other pathology.

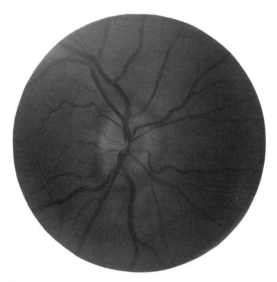

Figure 6.38 Early papilloedema (courtesy of Professor A.C. Bird)

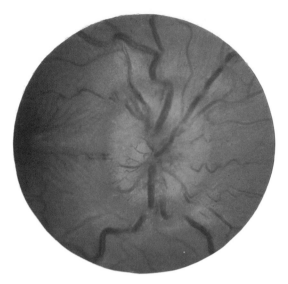

Figure 6.40 Advanced papilloedema with retinal folds (courtesy of Professor A.C. Bird)

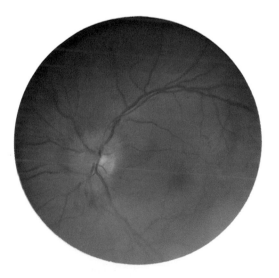

Figure 6.39 Established papilloedema

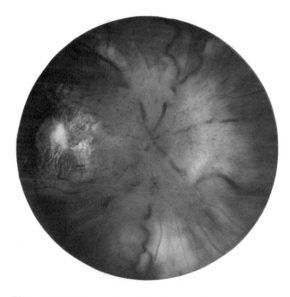

Figure 6.41 Advanced papilloedema with macular star

Signs

Early papilloedema

- Visual symptoms are absent.
- Visual acuity is normal.
- Optic disc shows hyperaemia and indistinctness of the superior, inferior and nasal disc margins, and blurring of peripapillary nerve fibre layer (Figure 6.38).
- Loss of previous spontaneous venous pulsation. However, because about 20% of normals do not show spontaneous venous pulsation, its absence does not necessarily mean that the intracranial pressure is raised. If venous pulsation is well preserved the diagnosis of papilloedema is unlikely.
- Blind spot is normal.

Established (fully developed) papilloedema

- Transient visual obscurations, lasting a few seconds, may occur on standing.
- Visual acuity may be normal or it may be reduced by macular oedema, haemorrhage or hard exudate.
- Optic disc shows venous engorgement, elevation of its surface, partial obscuration of the small traversing blood vessels and obliteration of the cup (Figure 6.39). The disc margin is indistinct and may be surrounded by peripapillary flame-shaped haemorrhages and cotton-wool spots. As the swelling increases, the optic nerve head appears to be enlarged and circumferential retinal folds may develop on its temporal side (Figure 6.40). Hard exudates may radiate from the centre of the fovea in the form of an incomplete star with its temporal part missing (Figure 6.41).
- Blind spot is enlarged.

Vintage papilloedema

- Visual acuity is variable.
- Optic disc takes on a champagne cork-like appearance without exudates and haemorrhages (Figure 6.42). This appearance indicates that the papilloedema has been present for several months.

Atrophic papilloedema

- Visual acuity is severely impaired.
- Optic disc is white and has indistinct margins due to gliosis (Figure 6.43). This appearance is also referred to as secondary optic atrophy and may be seen in patients with a history of cerebral tumours or treated benign intracranial hypertension.

Differential diagnosis

Pseudopapilloedema

Hypermetropia (long sight)   This may be associated with a rather small and crowded optic disc with a small or absent optic cup. However, venous pulsation should be present and the tiny blood vessels crossing the disc should appear uninterrupted.

Drusen (hyaline bodies)   Drusen of the optic disc are present in 1:300 of the population and are frequently familial. In children, when the drusen are buried within the substance of the optic nerve head, they may mimic early papilloedema (Figure 6.44). The main distinguishing features are:
- Absence of optic cup.
- Disc colour is pink or yellow.

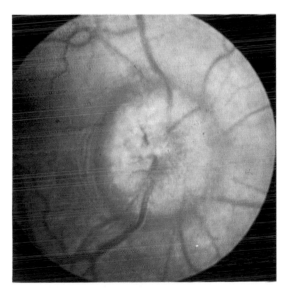

Figure 6.42 Vintage papilloedema (courtesy of Mr R. Marsh)

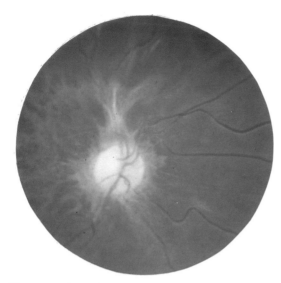

Figure 6.43 Secondary optic atrophy (courtesy of Mr E. Glover)

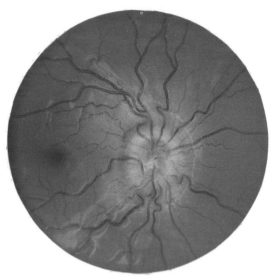

Figure 6.44 Pseudopapilloedema in a 12-year-old girl due to presumed buried drusen

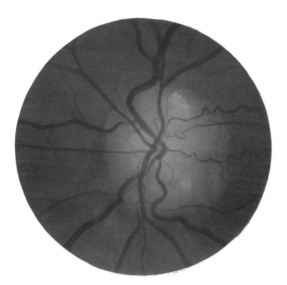

Figure 6.45 Exposed optic disc drusen (hyaline bodies)

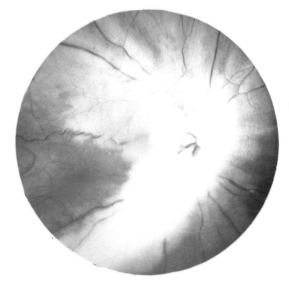

Figure 6.46 Myelinated retinal nerve fibres

- Disc margins may have a 'lumpy' appearance.
- Presence of anomalous and prematurely branching blood vessels emerging from the disc.
- Normal peripapillary retinal striations.

During the early teens the drusen gradually become exposed and appear as pearly irregularities on the disc surface (Figure 6.45).

Opaque nerve fibres These are usually unilateral and are characterized by a striking appearance of irregular white patches of myelinated retinal nerve fibres extending from the optic disc (Figure 6.46).

Disc swelling In general, unilateral cases of disc swelling should be considered to be due to one of the following causes.

- *Vascular*: central retinal vein occlusion (see Figure 3.7) and anterior ischaemic optic neuropathy (see Figure 3.11).
- *Inflammation*: optic papillitis (see Figure 6.7).
- *Compression*: optic nerve tumours and raised intraorbital pressure.
- *Infiltration*: granulomata (see Figure 7.11) and neoplastic lesions (see Figure 11.4).

Management

All patients with disc swelling, whether unilateral or bilateral, require urgent assessment. Referral should be by telephone and not just by letter.

- Unilateral cases should have an ophthalmological assessment first. If the diagnosis is not readily apparent, a CT or MR scan of the orbit may be required
- Bilateral cases are nearly always neurological and should be referred directly to a neurologist. After a careful clinical history and examination, CT or MR scanning is required in nearly every case.

Note: the most common cause of an intracranial tumour is a metastasis.

Benign intracranial hypertension

In a minority of patients with papilloedema no obvious structural abnormality is found, even after MRI scanning to exclude a posterior fossa lesion. A presumptive diagnosis of benign intracranial hypertension can be made. Many subjects are overweight women on the contraceptive pill.

- Treatment may include stopping 'the Pill', weight reduction, administration of a carbonic anhydrase inhibitor such as acetazolamide (Diamox) and repeated lumbar punctures.
- Lumbar puncture is safe in this situation despite raised intracranial pressure, because the brain is thought to be diffusely swollen and sudden dangerous intracranial shifts are unlikely. The only other clinical situation where a lumbar puncture is indicated in the presence of raised intracranial pressure and papilloedema is meningitis.
- Prognosis in most cases is good because the condition is self-limiting within a few months. The main danger is visual impairment due to secondary optic atrophy due to chronic papilloedema

Subarachnoid haemorrhage

Some patients develop multiple retinal and/or preretinal (subhyaloid) haemorrhages (Figure 6.47). Initially they are not associated with papilloedema although in about 20% mild papilloedema develops within several hours. Very occasionally, a large preretinal haemorrhage breaks through into the vitreous cavity (*Terson's syndrome*).

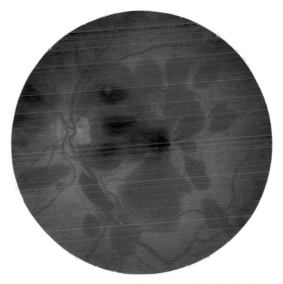

Figure 6.47 Large retinal and preretinal (subhyaloid) haemorrhages in a patient with an acute subarachnoid haemorrhage. Note the absence of papilloedema

Carotid–cavernous fistula

Definition

An arteriovenous fistula is an abnormal communication between arteries and veins. The blood within the affected vein becomes 'arterialized', the intravenous pressure rises and venous drainage may be altered in both rate and direction. In a carotid–cavernous fistula there is an abnormal communication between a branch of the carotid artery and the cavernous sinus. The two main types are *direct* and *indirect* (dural shunts). Each has different aetiologies and clinical features.

Direct fistula

Causes

In this type of fistula, the arterial blood passes directly through a defect in the wall of the intracavernous portion of the internal carotid artery.

- Head trauma (penetrating or non-penetrating) is responsible for 75% of cases. A basal skull fracture causes tearing of the internal carotid artery within the surrounding cavernous sinus. Traumatic fistulae are usually associated with high flow rates and severe symptoms.
- Spontaneous rupture of an intracavernous aneurysm or an atherosclerotic artery accounts

for the remaining 25%. Postmenopausal hypertensive women are at particular risk. These usually have lower flow rates and less severe features than traumatic fistulae.

Clinical features

These vary according to the size and location of the lesion. Because direct carotid–cavernous fistulae have a high flow of blood through them, the onset of symptoms is frequently sudden and dramatic. The signs are:

- Engorged episcleral and conjunctival blood vessels (Figure 6.48), and chemosis (Figure 6.49). In some cases the rise in episcleral venous pressure causes elevation of intraocular pressure (secondary glaucoma).
- Proptosis which is typically pulsatile; it is associated with both a bruit and a thrill which are abolished by ipsilateral carotid compression in the neck. A cephalic bruit may also be present.
- Ophthalmoplegia is very common and is caused primarily by involvement of the ocular motor nerves. The sixth nerve is involved in about 50% of patients with ophthalmoplegia, with variable involvement of the third and fourth nerves. Engorgement and enlargement of the extraocular muscles may also contribute to defective ocular mobility.
- Reduced visual acuity is common and may become permanent.

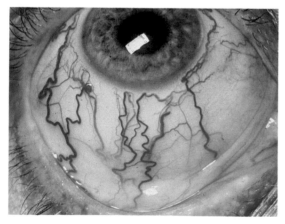

Figure 6.48 Grossly dilated conjunctival blood vessels in a patient with a carotid–cavernous fistula (courtesy of Professor A.C. Bird)

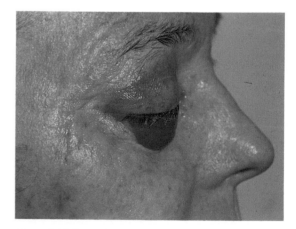

Figure 6.49 Gross chemosis in a patient with a carotid–cavernous fistula

- Fundus changes include vascular engorgement and central retinal vein occlusion (see Figure 3.7).
- Anterior segment ischaemia occurs in about 20% of cases. It is characterized by corneal epithelial oedema, aqueous flare and cells, iris atrophy, rubeosis and cataract.

Differential diagnosis

The clinical features may mimic thyroid eye disease, but in contrast to thyroid eye disease, fistulae are usually unilateral although occasionally bilateral features occur.

Treatment

Surgery may be indicated if spontaneous closure secondary to thrombosis of the cavernous sinus or its tributaries does not occur. Traumatic fistulae are less likely to close without treatment than spontaneous fistulae because of their higher flow.

The majority of carotid–cavernous fistulae are not life threatening and the major organ at risk is the eye. The main indications for surgery are:

- Visual deterioration due to glaucoma
- Diplopia.
- Intolerable bruit or headache.
- Severe exposure keratopathy due to proptosis.

Many methods aimed at obliteration of either the fistula, its afferent vessels or its efferent vessels have been tried. These include intravascular balloons via a catheter in the internal carotid artery and/or embolization with glue or particulate material.

Indirect fistula (dural shunt)

In this type of fistula, the intracavernous portion of the internal carotid artery remains intact, and arterial blood flows through the meningeal branches of the external or internal carotid arteries indirectly into the cavernous sinus. The main types are:

- Communication between the meningeal branches of the internal carotid artery and the cavernous sinus.

- Communication between the meningeal branches of the external carotid artery and the cavernous sinus.
- Communications from both the internal and external carotid arteries.

Causes

- Congenital – it is thought that in some cases the shunts are congenital malformations and that the onset of clinical features may be caused by intracranial venous thrombosis.
- Spontaneous rupture after minor trauma or straining, especially in a hypertensive patient.

Clinical features

Because indirect fistulae have a slow blood flow through them, the clinical features are much more subtle than in direct fistulae, so that they may be misdiagnosed or missed.

- Presentation in most patients is with mild proptosis, dilated episcleral vessels and raised intraocular pressure.
- Other features include pain, ptosis, ophthalmoplegia and a bruit.

Treatment

Most cases recover spontaneously without treatment. Surgical intervention may be required in a few.

Migraine
Definition

Migraine is a familial disorder characterized by recurrent attacks of headache widely variable in intensity, frequency and duration. Attacks are commonly unilateral and are associated with anorexia, nausea and vomiting. In some cases they are preceded by, or associated with, neurological and mood disturbances. However, all these characteristics are not necessarily present in each attack or in each patient. The main types of migraine are:

- Common.
- Classic.
- Focal.
- Migraine sine migraine.
- Retinal.
- Ophthalmoplegic.
- Complicated.
- Coital.
- Cluster.

Clinical features

Common migraine

In common migraine the headache is accompanied by autonomic nervous system dysfunction (e.g. pallor and nausea) but without other neurological features.

- Premonitory features include changes in mood, frequent yawning or other non-specific pro-dromal symptoms such as poor concentration.
- Headache starts anywhere on the cranium and is pounding or throbbing. It usually spreads to involve one half or the whole of the head. In some cases the pain is retro-orbital and may be mistaken for eye or sinus disease.
- During the attack, which lasts for hours to a day or more, the patient is frequently photophobic and seeks relief in a quiet dark environment or from sleep.

Because of the absence of the well-known migrainous visual distortions, severe nausea and vomiting, many patients with common migraine do not recognize that they have migraine.

Classic migraine

This type is less common but better recognized. The attack is heralded by a visual or sometimes an auditory aura which lasts between 15 and 45 minutes.

- Visual aura may consist of bright or dark spots, zig-zags, heat haze distortions, jig-saw puzzle effects, scintillating scotomata, tunnel vision, homonymous hemianopias, altitudinal hemianopias and fortification spectra. A fortification spectrum starts as a small bright positive paracentral scotoma lined on one side with luminous zig-zag lines (Figure 6.50a). After several minutes the fortification spectrum grad-ually enlarges with the open end pointing

centrally and often lined on the inner edge by an absent area of vision (negative scotoma) (Figure 6.50b). As the scotoma expands it may drift or march towards the temporal periphery before breaking up (Figure 6.50c,d). These features are said to be pathognomonic of migraine, but rarely they may be caused by degenerative arterial problems in the occipital poles.

- Headache is similar to that in common migraine but it may be absent, trivial or very severe, with considerable variation between attacks even in the same individual.

Focal migraine

In addition to the other symptoms of migraine the patient may develop transient dysphasia, hemisensory symptoms or even focal weakness.

Migraine sine migraine

This is characterized by episodic visual or other focal disturbances but without subsequent headache. Older patients with a past history of common or classic migraine are typically affected. Consider the possibility of transient ischaemic attacks.

Retinal migraine

This is characterized by acute but transient unilateral loss of vision which is identical to that seen in patients with amaurosis fugax (see Chapter 3). Ocular migraine may occasionally occur in middle-aged patients with no past history of migraine. It is prudent to investigate as if they were having attacks of amaurosis fugax.

Ophthalmoplegic migraine

This rare type of migraine typically starts before the age of 10 years. It is characterized by a transient third nerve palsy which begins after the headache is well established.

Complicated migraine

Rarely the focal neurological features fail to recover fully after the migraine attack is over and the patient is left with a hemisensory disturbance or partial visual field loss. Other neurological sequelae are exceptional.

Coital migraine

Here a sudden, severe headache occurs during sexual intercourse, typically at orgasm. It is excruciating for some minutes and then gradually declines. In these patients it is usually advisable to perform a CT scan or a lumbar puncture to exclude the possibility of a subarachnoid haemorrhage. Coital migraine tends to be self-limiting with headache becoming less prominent with subsequent 'performances'.

Cluster headaches

This is a migraine variant which typically affects males during the fourth and fifth decades of life. It is characterized by a typical, stereotyped headache accompanied by various autonomic phenomena occurring almost every day for a period of some weeks.

- Headache is unilateral, oculotemporal, excruciating, sharp and deep. It begins relatively

abruptly and decreases over a few minutes. It lasts between 10 minutes and 2 hours and then clears quickly. It may occur several times in a 24-hour period often at particular times, not infrequently at around 2 a.m. Once the 'cluster' is over there may be a long headache-free interval of several years.
- Autonomic phenomena associated with the headache include lacrimation, conjunctival injection and rhinorrhoea. Cluster headaches are also a common cause of a transient or permanent postganglionic Horner's syndrome.

Treatment of migraine

- General measures include elimination of conditions and agents that may precipitate an attack of migraine such as coffee, chocolate, alcohol, cheese, oral contraceptives, stress, lack of sleep and long intervals without food.

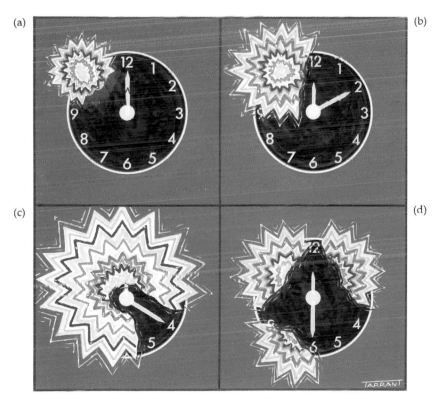

(a)   (b)   (c)   (d)

Figure 6.50 Progression of a classic migrainous scintillating scotoma and fortification spectrum

- Prophylaxis may be with β-adrenergic blockers, calcium channel blockers, amitriptyline, clonidine, pizotifen and low dose aspirin (150 mg/day).
- Treatment of an acute attack can be with ergotamine tartrate, non-steroidal anti-inflammatory agents, paracetamol or codeine analogues. An antiemetic by mouth, suppository or injection may also be useful.

Wilson's disease

Definition

Wilson's disease is a rare autosomal recessive disorder caused by a deficiency of the plasma copper-carrying protein caeruloplasmin. It is characterized by widespread deposition of copper in the tissues with particular impact on the liver and brain.

Systemic features

Wilson's disease becomes manifest in three main ways.

1. *Hepatic*: this may present as acute hepatitis, cirrhosis or hepatosplenomegaly (e.g. on screening siblings).
2. *Neurological*: involvement of the basal ganglia may cause involuntary movements, rigidity, tremor or even a flap with dysarthria and dysphagia. There is also evidence of intellectual decline.
3. *Psychiatric*: this may be manifest as manic-depression, bizarre behaviour disorders or even a schizophrenic-like illness.

The only difficulty with diagnosing Wilson's disease is remembering to consider it as a possibility.

Ocular features

- Kayser–Fleischer ring is present in virtually all cases. It consists of copper granules located deep in the cornea at the periphery of Descemet's membrane (Figure 6.51). The ring is more pronounced in the vertical meridians of the cornea and it may disappear when the patient is treated with penicillamine. Patients suspected to be suffering from Wilson's disease should be referred to an ophthalmologist because the Kayser–Fleischer ring is not usually evident to the naked eye but can be detected by slit lamp examination.
- Green 'sunflower' cataract is less common.

Diagnostic tests

- Serum ceruloplasmin assay is the definitive diagnostic test.
- Urinary copper excretion is high.
- Liver biopsy shows excess copper and evidence of cirrhosis.

Treatment

Treatment with the chelating agent D-penicillamine is not without potential problems and patients require regular haematological and biochemical screening tests. In a minority of patients the drug causes nephrotic syndrome, myasthenia or an SLE-like illness.

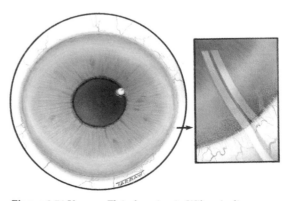

Figure 6.51 Kayser–Fleischer ring in Wilson's disease

Esssential blepharospasm

Clinical features

Essential blepharospasm is an involuntary idiopathic spasm of the orbicularis muscle. In severe cases it may be very distressing because it may make the patient temporarily blind. The condition should be differentiated from hemifacial spasm and apraxia of lid opening.

Treatment

Mild cases can be treated by muscle relaxants and facial nerve blocks. In severe cases the injection of botulinum toxin into the orbicularis muscle may be most helpful

Further reading

BASKIN, D.S. and WILSON, C.B. (1986) Surgical management of craniopharyngioma: A review of 74 cases. *Journal of Neurology*, **65**, 22–27

FISHER, C.M. (1980) Late-life migraine accompaniments as a cause of unexplained transient ischaemic attacks. *Canadian Journal of Neurological Science*, **45**, 63–67

FLEISHMAN, J.A., BECK, R.W., LINARES, O.A. *et al*. (1987) Deficits in visual function after resolution of optic neuritis. *Ophthalmology*, **94**, 1029–1035

HENNEKEN, A.M., MILLER, N.R., DEBRUN, G.M. *et al*. (1989) Treatment of carotid-cavernous fistulas using a detachable balloon catheter through the superior ophthalmic vein. *Archives of Ophthalmology*, **107**, 87–92

HUPP, S.L., KLINE, L.B. and CORBETT, J.J. (1989) Visual disturbances in migraine. *Survey of Ophthalmology*, **33**, 221–236

JACOBS, L., KINKEL, P.R. and KINKEL, W.R. (1986) Silent brain lesions in patients with isolated idiopathic optic neuritis. *Archives of Neurology*, **43**, 452–455

JOHNS, R., LAVIN, P., ELLIOT, J.H. *et al*. (1986) Magnetic resonance imaging of the brain in isolated optic neuritis. *Archives of Ophthalmology*, **104**, 1486–1488

JOHNSON, L.N., HEPLER, R.S., YEE, R.D. *et al*. (1986) Magnetic resonance imaging in craniopharyngioma. *American Journal of Ophthalmology*, **102**, 242–244

KELTNER, J.L., SATTERFIELD, D., DUBLIN, A.B. *et al*. (1987) Dural and carotid cavernous fistulas. Diagnosis, management, and complications. *Ophthalmology*, **94**, 1585–1600

KURTZE, J.F. (1985) Optic neuritis or multiple sclerosis. *Archives of Neurology*, **42**, 704–710

LEWIS, R.A., VIJAYAN, N., WATSON, C. *et al*. (1989) Visual field loss in migraine. *Ophthalmology*, **96**, 321–326

ORCUTT, J.C., PAGE, N.G. and SANDERS, M.D. (1984) Factors affecting visual loss in benign intracranial hypertension. *Ophthalmology*, **91**, 1303–1312

REPKA, M.X., MILLER, N.R. and MILLER, N. (1989) Visual outcome after surgical removal of craniopharyngiomas. *Ophthalmology*, **96**, 195–199

RIZZO, J.F. and LESSELL, S. (1988) Risk of developing multiple sclerosis after uncomplicated optic neuritis. A long term prospective study. *Neurology*, **38**, 185–190

SANDERS, M.D. and SENNEHENN, R.H. (1980) Differential diagnosis of optic disc oedema. *Transactions of the Ophthalmological Society of the United Kingdom*, **100**, 123–131

SAVINO, P.J., GLASER, J.S. and ROSENBERG, M.A. (1979) A clinical analysis of pseudopapilloedema *Archives of Ophthalmology*, **97**, 71–75

SPOOR, T.C. and ROCKWELL, D.L. (1988) Treatment of optic neuritis with intravenous megadose corticosteroids. *Ophthalmology*, **95**, 131–134

WATERS, W.E. and O'CONNOR, P.J. (1975) Prevalence of migraine. *Journal of Neurology, Neurosurgery and Psychiatry*, **38**, 613–616

YOUNG, I.R., HALL, A.S., PALLIS, C.A. *et al*. (1981) Nuclear magnetic resonance imaging of the brain in multiple sclerosis. *Lancet*, **i**, 1063–1066

7

Pulmonary disorders

Sarcoidosis

Definition

Sarcoidosis is a common multisystem disorder of unknown aetiology characterized by the presence of non-caseating granulomata in the lungs and other organs. The condition is more common in Blacks than in Whites.

Systemic features

Presentation

This is usually in one of two ways:

1. During the third decade with an acute onset characterized by erythema nodosum, parotid enlargement and hilar lymphadenopathy.
2. During the fifth decade with an insidious onset characterized by fatigue, dyspnoea and arthralgia.

Signs

- The lungs are involved in between 85% and 95% of patients.
- Skin lesions include erythema nodosum (Figure 7.1) and a variety of other infiltrative lesions.
- A transient polyarthritis or a chronic arthritis can occur. In some patients the disease causes destructive cystic bony lesions, predominantly around the wrists and ankle joints.
- Central nervous system involvement may cause: cranial nerve palsies, peripheral neuropathy, granulomatous meningitis and mononeuritis multiplex.

- Cardiomyopathy with granulomatous involvement of the His-Purkinje system may cause arrhythmias and conduction defects, and occasionally sudden death.
- Renal disease may be secondary to granulomatous infiltration or hypercalcaemia.
- Liver disease
- Lymphadenopathy and hepatosplenomegaly.

Diagnostic tests

Although the diagnosis is often easy, in some patients many of the features may be missing and the following special investigations may be useful.

Chest X-ray

Over 90% of patients with ocular sarcoid will have an abnormal chest X-ray. The X-ray changes can be divided into the following four stages.

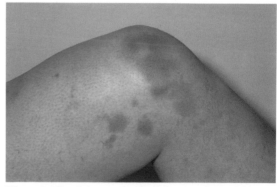

Figure 7.1 Erythema nodosum in acute sarcoidosis

98

Stage 1 This consists of bilateral hilar lymphadenopathy and normal lung parenchyma (Figure 7.2).

Stage 2 This is characterized by bilateral hilar lymphadenopathy and the appearance of reticulonodular infiltrates.

Stage 3 This is characterized by reticulonodular infiltration only (Figure 7.3).

Stage 4 This is characterized by progressive pulmonary fibrosis.

Biopsy

- Transbronchial lung biopsy via a fibreoptic bronchoscope is accurate in about 90% of active cases.
- Lacrimal gland biopsy by a transconjunctival route may be considered in patients with suspected sarcoidosis, particularly if the lacrimal glands are enlarged or if they demonstrate increased gallium uptake. Biopsies are positive in 25% of patients with unenlarged glands and in 75% with lacrimal gland enlargement.
- Biopsy of conjunctiva, lymph node, tonsil and liver may also give histological confirmation.

Kveim–Siltzbach test

This test relies on the fact that a saline suspension of sarcoid tissue (antigen), obtained from the spleen of a patient with sarcoidosis, and introduced intradermally, induces a granuloma of sarcoid type. The test is positive in 85–90% of patients with early or active disease but this sensitivity decreases with chronicity. False positives can occur in other granulomatous conditions such as Crohn's disease and tuberculosis. It is vital that well-validated Kveim material is used. Extreme care must be taken to avoid simultaneous inoculation of foreign body material which may induce a non-specific granulomatous reaction. The skin site is then biopsied at 4–6 weeks whether or not a palpable papule is present. The specimen is then examined histologically.

Mantoux test

Although the Mantoux test is negative in a very high percentage of patients with sarcoidosis, it is now of limited diagnostic value except in areas with a high incidence of positive tuberculin tests.

Serum angiotensin converting enzyme

Angiotensin converting enzyme (ACE) is produced by many cells in the body. Normal serum levels of ACE are 12–35 nmol/min per µl in men and 11–29 nmol/min per µl in women. Serum ACE is usually elevated in patients with active sarcoidosis and is normal during remissions. The test has specificity deficiencies because the serum ACE level may be raised in other conditions such as tuberculosis, carcinomatosis, histoplasmosis, rheumatoid arthritis and ankylosing spondylitis, some of which may be associated with uveitis. In patients with suspected neurosarcoid CSF, ACE should be measured.

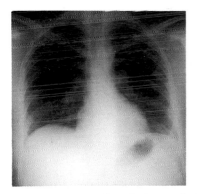

Figure 7.2 Bilateral lymphadenopathy in acute (stage 1) sarcoidosis (courtesy of Dr M. Smith)

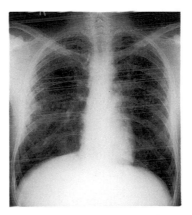

Figure 7.3 Reticulonodular infiltration in stage 3 sarcoidosis (courtesy of Dr M. Smith)

Calcium assays

Calcium metabolism is abnormal in sarcoidosis. Hypercalciuria is common but hypercalcaemia is unusual.

Gallium-67 scan

Gallium scan of the head, neck and thorax frequently shows increased uptake in patients with active sarcoidosis because the gallium is taken up by mitotically active liposomes of granulocytes. This is an interesting research tool and shows some correlation with disease activity. However, it has no place in the routine diagnosis and management of sarcoidosis.

Bronchoalveolar lavage

There is considerable interest in the alterations in immune responses in patients with sarcoidosis. The technique of bronchoalveolar lavage allows direct sampling of bronchoalveolar cell populations and in most series has shown a raised proportion of activated T-helper lymphocytes. This is in sharp contrast to the reactive anergy shown in delayed hypersensitivity skin tests (e.g. Mantoux test). However, the results are not consistent or specific enough to be of routine diagnostic use.

Treatment and prognosis

- Acute sarcoidosis may require no specific treatment as the disease may regress spontaneously within 2 years and usually does not recur.
- Chronic sarcoidosis may require systemic steroids in order to prevent serious disability and even death from respiratory failure.
- Specific indications for systemic steroids are: progressive deterioration of pulmonary function, central nervous system involvement, hypercalcaemia and severe ocular disease.

Ocular features

The eye is involved in about 25% of patients. Ocular involvement may occur in patients with few, if any, systemic symptoms, as well as in those with inactive systemic disease, and the diagnosis may be missed. In acute sarcoidosis, the ocular inflammation is frequently unilateral and, as the disease becomes chronic, bilateral involvement is the rule. Most anterior segment complications (Figure 7.4) respond to topical steroids, although systemic steroids may be required in patients with severe involvement of the posterior segment.

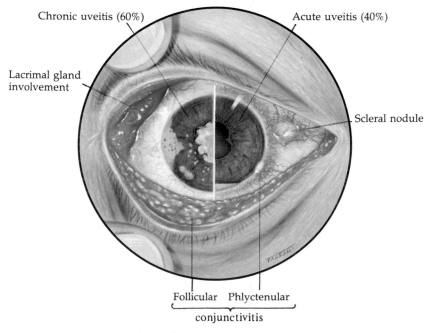

Chronic uveitis (60%)   Acute uveitis (40%)

Lacrimal gland involvement

Scleral nodule

Follicular   Phlyctenular
conjunctivitis

Figure 7.4 Anterior segment complications of sarcoidosis

External

- Eyelid involvement is uncommon and may consist of violaceous sarcoid plaques (*lupus pernio*) (Figure 7.5) or lid granulomata which may be mistaken for small chalazia.
- Conjunctival granulomata which may be suitable for diagnostic biopsy are uncommon. Phlyctens are very rare.
- Lacrimal gland infiltration is uncommon but, when severe, it may be responsible for keratoconjunctivitis sicca. Rarely, extralacrimal orbital involvement may also occur.

Anterior uveitis

Anterior uveitis is by far the most common complication and, in fact, sarcoidosis is responsible for about 5% of all cases of anterior uveitis in the UK. The uveitis is of two types.

Acute anterior uveitis This is unilateral and non-granulomatous and occurs in young patients with acute sarcoid. The long-term prognosis is usually good.

Chronic anterior uveitis This is more common than the acute type. It is usually bilateral, granulomatous and occurs in older patients with chronic lung disease (Figures 7.6 and 7.7).

Posterior segment

The posterior segment is involved in about 7% of patients with chronic sarcoidosis and in 25% of patients with ocular sarcoid. The fundus changes are caused by granulomatous involvement of the retinal veins, the vitreous, the choroid and the optic nerve head (Figure 7.8).

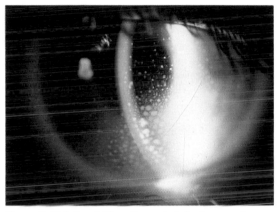

Figure 7.6 Mutton fat keratic precipitates in granulomatous anterior uveitis associated with chronic sarcoidosis

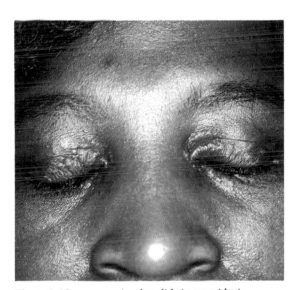

Figure 7.5 Lupus pernio of eyelids in sarcoidosis

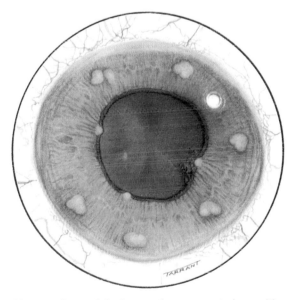

Figure 7.7 Iris nodules in granulomatous anterior uveitis associated with chronic sarcoidosis

Retinal vasculitis   Retinal vasculitis involving the retinal veins (periphlebitis), characterized by perivenous cuffing of peripheral retinal veins, is the most frequent finding.

- In mild cases only a few segments are involved.
- Advanced periphlebitis is characterized by 'candlewax drippings' due to perivascular accumulation of granulomatous tissue (Figure 7.9).
- Acute sarcoid retinopathy, which is rare, is characterized by vitreous haze, severe periphlebitis and haemorrhages (Figure 7.10).

Neovascularization   New vessel formation on the retina and optic nerve head is usually secondary to wide areas of capillary non-perfusion in some patients with acute sarcoid retinopathy or retinal branch vein occlusion.

Vitreous   Vitreous involvement may consist of a diffuse haze or opacities either of the 'string of pearls' type or small 'cotton balls' which lie on the surface of the inferior retina anterior to the equator (Lander's sign).

Choroid   Involvement of the choroid is of two types.

1. Multiple, small, deep-yellow choroidal lesions associated with mottling of the retinal pigment epithelium are the most common.

2. Large, solitary, choroidal granulomata are rare and may be mistaken for choroidal tumours.

Optic nerve   Granulomata of the optic nerve are uncommon (Figure 7.11).

Tuberculosis

Definition

Tuberculosis (TB) is a chronic granulomatous infection caused by either bovine or human tubercle bacilli. The former causes TB through the drinking of milk from infected cattle and the latter is spread by 'droplet infection'.

Systemic features

Primary TB

This occurs in subjects not previously exposed to the bacillus. It typically causes the 'primary complex' in the chest (Ghon focus + regional lymphadenopathy) which usually heals spontaneously and causes little if any systemic symptoms.

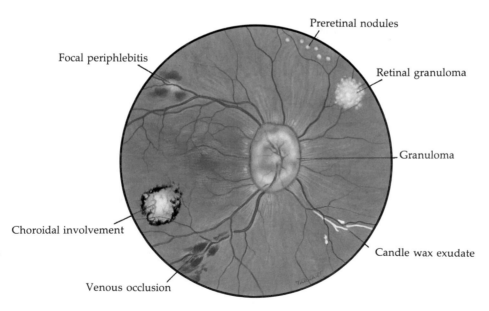

Figure 7.8 Posterior segment complications of sarcoidosis

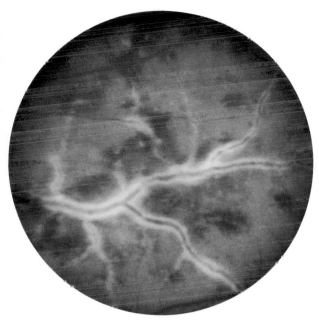

Figure 7.9 Severe retinal periphlebitis in sarcoidosis

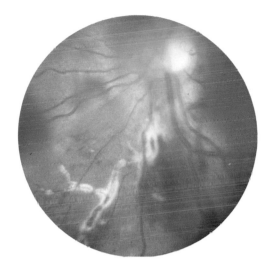

Figure 7.10 Severe retinal periphlebitis with 'candlewax drippings' and vitreous haemorrhage in sarcoidosis. (courtesy of Mr J. Shilling)

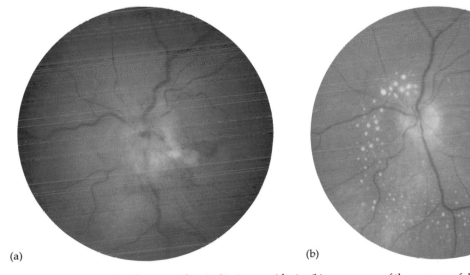

(a)

(b)

Figure 7.11 (a) Severe involvement of optic disc in sarcoidosis; (b) appearance of the same eye following treatment with systemic steroids showing small residual retinal nodules

Postprimary TB

This is due to reinfection or, rarely, recrudescence of a primary lesion, usually in a patient with impaired immunity as from diabetes, systemic steroid therapy, old age or malnutrition. The clinical features include fibrocaseous pulmonary lesions and miliary TB from haematogenous spread. Theoretically, seeding of the uvea by live bacilli may occur during the primary and miliary stages giving rise to either caseating nodules or small miliary tubercules.

Treatment

Treatment is generally straightforward. In pulmonary and glandular TB, short course quadruple chemotherapy is with rifampicin and isoniazid for a total of 6 months combined with ethambutol and pyrazinamide for the first 2 months. For TB involving other sites rifampicin and isoniazid are usually continued for 9–12 months. It is imperative that a patient with TB involving any site should be notified to the Department of Public Health so that contact tracing can be initiated. The prognosis is excellent with cure rates in excess of 97% if the organism is sensitive.

Ocular features

There is no specific finding in ocular TB and the clinical picture is pleomorphic. As in sarcoidosis, virtually any ocular and periocular structure can be involved including the orbit, skin, conjunctiva, cornea and uvea.

Uveitis

In the UK, TB is a rare cause of uveitis accounting for less than 1% of all cases. Despite this it is important not to miss the diagnosis because it is one of the few uveal inflammations which can be cured with antibiotics. The diagnosis of ocular TB is always presumptive and is based on indirect evidence such as:

- Intractable steroid-resistant uveitis.
- Negative findings for other causes of uveitis.
- Positive findings for systemic TB.
- Positive response to isoniazid therapy of 300 mg/day for 3 weeks.

Anterior uveitis due to TB is characteristically granulomatous and may resemble that associated with sarcoidosis. Choroidal involvement may be unifocal or multifocal. Rarely, a large solitary choroidal granuloma may be mistaken for a tumour.

TB uveitis is treated with quadruple chemotherapy for 12 months.

Wegener's granulomatosis

Definition

Wegener's granulomatosis is a rare idiopathic disease characterized by granulomatous inflammation and necrosis of the respiratory tract and other organs. The disease affects males more commonly than females. A high proportion of patients are positive for antineutrophilic cytoplasmic antibodies.

Systemic features

Wegener's disease most commonly presents during the fourth and fifth decades with initially mild upper respiratory tract symptoms accompanied by night sweats or arthralgia. Fulminating cases may present with rapidly progressive renal failure.

Upper respiratory tract

The upper respiratory tract mucosa is involved in about 90% of cases. Subsequent involvement of the underlying cartilage and bone by the necrotizing process may lead to the following complications:

- Perforation of the nasal septum.
- Destruction of the bones of the paranasal sinuses.
- Collapse of the nasal arch resulting in a 'saddle nose' deformity.
- Nasal–paranasal sinus fistulae.

Lower respiratory tract

The lower resiratory tract is involved in 90% of cases and is characterized by discrete, usually bilateral, pulmonary granulomata which may cause a productive cough and haemoptysis.

Miscellaneous

- A progressive glomerulonephritis may occur late in the course of the disease and is a common cause of death.
- Arthralgia is present in 50% of cases.
- Haemorrhagic dermatitis is common.
- Polyneuritis.
- Other organs that may be involved by a focal vasculitis include the spleen, heart and adrenal glands.

Treatment

Treatment is with systemic steroids and cyclophosphamide. The prognosis for life is variable.

Ocular features

About 30% of patients have ocular involvement which may be either primary or secondary to contiguous spread from the paranasal sinuses.

Anterior segment

- Peripheral ulcerative keratitis is the most serious complication (see Figure 5.4).
- Necrotizing scleritis similar to that seen in rheumatoid arthritis is common (see Figure 4.6).
- Conjunctivitis and episcleritis may also occur.

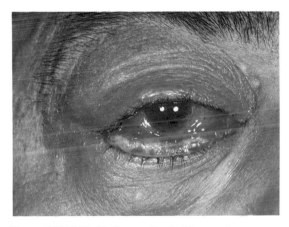

Figure 7.12 Orbital inflammation in Wegener's granulomatosis

Orbit

Orbital involvement is common and is the result of direct spread from diseased contiguous paranasal sinuses. The clinical features are those of a bilateral 'pseudotumour' characterized by pain and proptosis which may be associated with chemosis (Figure 7.12), ophthalmoplegia, congestion of the retinal vessels and disc oedema.

Posterior segment

- Retinal vasculitis leading to either focal retinal infarcts or major vascular occlusions is uncommon.
- Anterior ischaemic optic neuropathy is uncommon (see Figure 3.11).

Further reading

ADRAMS, J. and SCHLAEGEL, T.F. JR (1982) The role of the isoniazid therapeutic test in tuberculous uveitis. *American Journal of Ophthalmology*, **94**, 511–515

BAARSMA, G.S., LA HEY, F , GLAUSIUS, E. *et al.* (1987) The predictive value of serum angiotensin converting enzyme and lysozyme levels in the diagnosis of ocular sarcoidosis. *American Journal of Ophthalmology*, **104**, 211–217.

COLLINSON, J.M.T., MILLER, N.R. and GREEN, W.R. (1986) Involvement of orbital tissues in sarcoidosis. *American Journal of Ophthalmology*, **102**, 302–307.

D'CRUZ, D.P., BAGULEY, E., ASHERSON, R.A. *et al.* (1989) Ear, nose, and throat symptoms in subacute Wegener's granulomatosis. *British Journal of Medicine*, **299**, 419–422

DUKER, J.S., BROWN, G.C. and McNAMARA, J.A. (1988) Proliferative sarcoid retinopathy. *Ophthalmology*, **95**, 1680–1688.

JABS, D.A. and JOHNS, C.J. (1986) Ocular involvement in chronic sarcoidosis. *American Journal of Ophthalmology*, **102**, 297–301.

KARMA, A., HUHTI, E. and POUKKULA, A. A. (1988) Course and outcome of ocular sarcoidosis. *American Journal of Ophthalmology*, **106**, 467–472.

KARMA, A., POUKKULA, A. A. and RUOKONEN, A.O. (1987) Assessment of activity of ocular sarcoidosis by gallium scanning. *British Journal of Ophthalmology*, **71**, 361–367.

ROBIN, J.B., SCHANZLIN, D.J., MEISLER, D.M. *et al.* (1985) Ocular involvement in the respiratory vasculitides. *Survey of Ophthalmology*, **30**, 127–140

SANDERS, M.D. (1987) Duke-Elder Lecture. Retinal arteritis, retinal vasculitis and autoimmune retinal vasculitis. *Eye*, **1**, 441–465

SANDERS, M.D. and SHILLING, J.S. (1975) Retinal, choroidal,

and optic disc involvement in sarcoidosis. *Transactions of the Ophthalmological Society of the United Kingdom*, **96**, 140–144.

SPALTON, D.J. and SANDERS, M.D. (1981) Fundus changes in histologically confirmed sarcoidosis. *British Journal of Ophthalmology*, **65**, 348–358.

STONE, L.S. and EHRENBERG, M. (1984) Bilateral nodular sarcoid choroiditis with vitreous haemorrhage. *British Journal of Ophthalmology*, **68**, 660–666.

WEINREB, R.N. and TESSLER, H. (1984) Laboratory diagnosis of ophthalmic sarcoidosis. *Survey of Ophthalmology*, **28**, 653–664.

8

Gastrointestinal disorders

Crohn's disease

Definition

Crohn's disease (regional ileitis) is an idiopathic, chronic, relapsing disease characterized by multi-focal non-caseating granulomatous inflammation of the bowel which is characteristically transmural. The prevalence of HLA-B27 is high in patients with Crohn's disease, particularly when it is associated with arthritis.

Systemic features

Gastrointestinal

Involvement of the small bowel and the terminal ileum is most typically encountered. Perirectal complications such as fistulae, abscesses and fissures are also common. Other parts of the gastrointestinal tract that may also be involved are the oropharynx, oesophagus, stomach and the jejunum.

Extraintestinal

These include low-grade fever, weight loss, arthritis, psoriasis, erythema nodosum, and liver and kidney disease.

Ocular features

About 5% of cases have a variety of usually innocuous eye lesions.

- Conjunctivitis and anterior uveitis are the most common.

- Uncommon lesions are scleritis, keratitis, kerato-conjunctivitis sicca, orbital pseudotumour, choroiditis, retinal vasculitis and optic neuritis.

Ulcerative colitis

Definition

Ulcerative colitis is an uncommon, idiopathic, chronic, relapsing disease involving the rectum and extending for a variable distance proximally, occasionally to involve the entire colon. The disease is characterized by diffuse surface ulcera-tion of the gut mucosa with the development of crypt abscesses and pseudopolyposis. Females are affected more commonly than males.

Systemic features

Gastrointestinal

Presentation is usually during the second and third decades with bloody diarrhoea, anaemia, weight loss, fever, abdominal cramping pain, and nocturnal passing of small amounts of blood and mucus. Patients with long-standing disease are at increased risk of developing carcinoma of the colon.

Extraintestinal

These include erythema nodosum, liver disease and arthritis. The latter may affect either the large peripheral joints or it may be sarcoiliitis. Patients with arthritis have an increased prevalence of HLA-B27

Ocular features

- Acute anterior uveitis occurs in some patients and the attacks may be synchronized with exacerbation of colitis. Patients with associated sacroiliitis are at increased risk of developing uveitis.
- Optic papillitis is rare.

Whipple's disease

Definition

Whipple's disease is a very rare, idiopathic, multisystem disorder characterized by intestinal malabsorption and steatorrhoea. It affects males more commonly than females. The diagnosis is usually made by jejunal biopsy which demonstrates the presence of PAS-positive intracellular granules in macrophages (PAS = periodic acid–Schiff).

Systemic features

Gastrointestinal

Presentation is typically in the fifth decade with diarrhoea, abdominal pain, fever and weight loss.

Extraintestinal

These include arthralgia, hypermelanosis, peripheral lymphadenopathy, and occasionally neurological lesions and heart murmurs.

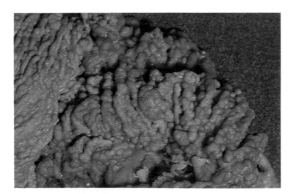

Figure 8.1 Familial polyposis coli

Ocular features

- Chronic anterior uveitis.
- Vitritis.
- Diffuse chorioretinitis.

Treatment with antibiotics is beneficial for both the systemic and ocular lesions.

Familial polyposis coli

Definition

Familial polyposis coli is a rare dominantly inherited condition characterized by multiple polyps of the colon.

Systemic features

Hundreds and sometimes thousands of adenomatous polyps are present throughout the entire colon (Figure 8.1). The polyps start to develop in adolescence and virtually all patients develop carcinoma of the colon by the age of 50. A total colectomy should therefore be carried out early in adult life in affected persons. Because of the dominant inheritance pattern, an intensive survey

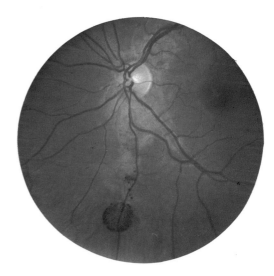

Figure 8.2 Hypertrophy of the retinal pigment epithelium in familial polyposis coli

of family members must be conducted. Unfortunately there is no phenotype biochemical abnormality or serological marker that indicates whether a family member will be affected by the disease.

Ocular features

Patients with polyposis coli frequently show patches of congenital hypertrophy of the retinal pigment epithelium (Figure 8.2). The presence of this condition in family members should arouse suspicion that the patient is at risk of polyposis coli.

Further reading

BAILLIE, J. and SOLTIS, R.D. (1985) Systemic complications of inflammatory bowel disease. *Geriatrics*, **40**, 53

CHAPMAN, P.D., CHURCH, W., BURN, J. *et al.* (1989) Congenital hypertrophy of the retinal pigment epithelium: a sign of familial adenomatous polyposis, *British Medical Journal*, **298**, 353 354

DUKER, J.S., BROWN, G.C. and BROOKS, L. (1987) Retinal vasculitis in Crohn's disease. *American Journal of Ophthalmology*, **103**, 664–668

LLOPIS, M.D. and MENEZO, J.L. (1987) Congenital hypertrophy of the retinal pigment epithelium and familial polyposis coli. *American Journal of Ophthalmology*, **103**, 235.

PETRILLI, E.A., McKINLEY, M. and TRONCALE, F.J. (1982) Ocular manifestations of inflammatory bowel disease. *Annals of Ophthalmology*, **14**, 356

SEDGWICK, L.A., KLINGELE, T.C., BURDE, R.M. *et al.* (1984) Optic neuritis in inflammatory bowel disease. *Journal of Clinical Neurology and Ophthalmology*, **4**, 3

WEINSTEIN, J.M., KOCH, K. and LANE, S. (1984) Orbital pseudotumour in Crohn's colitis. *Annals of Ophthalmology*, **16**, 278

ZAIDMAN, G.W. and COLES, R.S. (1981) Peripheral uveitis and ulcerative colitis. *Annals of Ophthalmology*, **16**, 275

9

Sexually transmitted diseases

Acquired immune deficiency syndrome

Definition

The acquired immune deficiency syndrome (AIDS) is defined as the occurrence of opportunistic infections, Kaposi's sarcoma (or other neoplasia) or both in patients who are not immunocompromised as a result of some other cause such as leukaemia or immunosuppressive therapy. The causative pathogen of AIDS is the human immunodeficiency virus (HIV) which is transmitted predominantly by sexual intercourse. Homosexual men are more commonly infected than heterosexuals. The virus may also be transmitted via contaminated blood to haemophiliacs and also to intravenous drug abusers by the sharing of syringes. Patients can be HIV positive and infective some years before they develop AIDS. The disease is invariably fatal.

Systemic features

Opportunistic infections

In the UK, AIDS patients will have one of the following diseases categorized by micro-organisms.

- *Protozoa*: *Pneumocystis carinii* pneumonia or disseminated disease, toxoplasmosis and cryptosporidiosis.
- *Viruses*: cytomegalovirus (CMV) retinitis, pneumonitis and colitis, and persistently invasive lesions due to herpes simplex.
- *Fungi*: cryptococcosis and oesophageal candidiasis.
- *Bacteria*: atypical mycobacteria and extrapulmonary tuberculosis.

Neoplasia

- Kaposi's sarcoma is a multifocal neoplasm of vascular origin that can present in an atypically aggressive form in AIDS patients. The tumour may affect the skin (Figure 9.1), mucous membranes and inside visceral organs.
- Lymphomas.

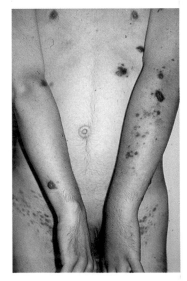

Figure 9.1 Cutaneous Kaposi's sarcoma (courtesy of Mr R. Marsh)

Ocular features

Ocular complications eventually affect about 75% of patients with AIDS

Kaposi's sarcoma

The conjunctiva and eyelids may be the earliest sites for the tumour.

- Conjunctival Kaposi's sarcoma appears as a bright red mass, most frequently in the lower fornix. Very early lesions may be mistaken for a subconjunctival haemorrhage (see Figure 11.2).
- Eyelid Kaposi's sarcoma appears as an elevated, non-tender purple nodule.

Herpes zoster ophthalmicus

Severe involvement by herpes zoster ophthalmicus can sometimes be the presenting manifestation of AIDS (Figure 9.2). The anterior uveitis associated with herpes zoster tends to be severe and prolonged. Herpes zoster affecting other parts of the body is also very common.

CMV retinitis

CMV retinitis is the most frequent opportunistic infection involving the eye in AIDS. It occurs in up to 45% of cases during the average 20-month course of survival of the AIDS patient. The retinitis is frequently bilateral and, if untreated, often leads to blindness. The appearance of CMV retinitis is a sign of systemic CMV infection and signifies profound suppression of immunity and a grave prognosis for life – most patients are dead within a few months. The clinical appearance of CMV retinitis is variable.

- Cotton-wool spots, identical to those seen in hypertension and diabetes, are frequently the initial lesions (see Figure 1.13). They are usually transient and resolve over a period of 4-6 weeks. Some patients also develop scattered retinal nerve fibre haemorrhages, usually in the absence of the cotton-wool spots.
- Central retinitis is characterized by a dense, white, well-demarcated area of retinal necrosis which frequently develops along the vascular arcades (Figure 9.3). Retinal haemorrhages may be present either within the area of retinitis or along its leading edge.
- Peripheral retinitis has a more granular, less intense, white appearance and is less well demarcated (Figure 9.4). It is more common than the central type although in many patients the two forms coexist.

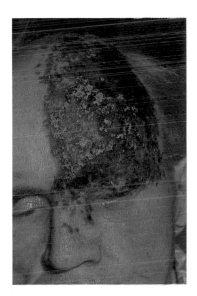

Figure 9.2 Very severe herpes zoster ophthalmicus

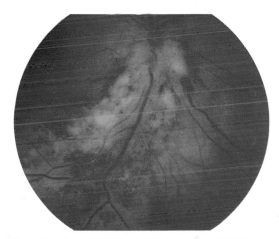

Figure 9.3 Central CMV retinitis (courtesy of Mr R. Marsh)

Irrespective of whether the retinitis starts centrally or in the periphery, it spreads slowly and relentlessly along the course of the blood vessels (Figure 9.5) and leads to retinal atrophy and, occasionally, also to involvement of the optic nerve head.

Treatment of CMV retinitis

- Ganciclovir (dihydroxypropoxymethylguanine) is presently first-line therapy. It is given intravenously 5 mg/kg twice daily for 10–20 days. There is a high risk of bone marrow suppression and care is necessary when other myelosuppressive therapy is being given, e.g. zidovudine (AZT). Intravitreal ganciclovir can be used if systemic therapy has failed.
- Foscarnet (phosphonoformate) is active against all herpes viruses and can also be used to treat CMV retinitis.

Miscellaneous retinitides

- Toxoplasmosis (see Figure 1.11).
- Candidiasis.
- Herpes simplex.
- Atypical mycobacteria.

They all require treatment with the appropriate antimicrobial agent.

Neuro-ophthalmic lesions

- Intracranial infection by pathogens such as *Cryptococcus neoformans* and *Toxoplasma gondii* may cause ocular motor nerve palsies, pupillary abnormalities, visual field defects and optic neuropathy.
- HIV may cause an encephalopathy with progressive dementia.

Acquired syphilis

Definition

Acquired syphilis is a sexually acquired infection with the spirochaete, *Treponema pallidum*. It is a systemic disease which, when untreated, has overt and covert stages.

Systemic features

Primary stage

This typically develops 9–90 days following exposure and is characterized by a painless ulcer (chancre) at the site of infection with associated

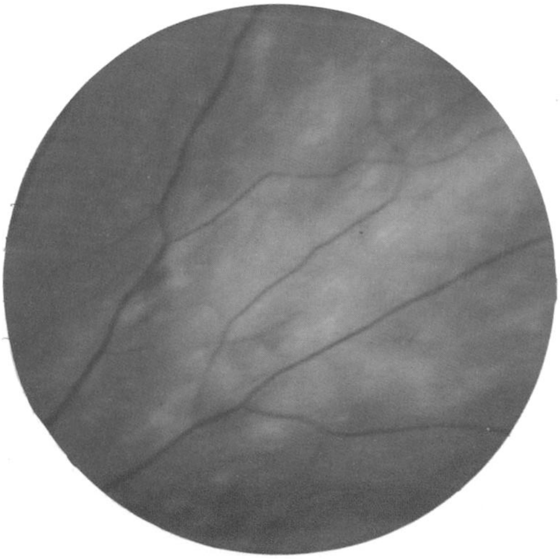

Figure 9.4 Peripheral CMV retinitis (courtesy of Mr D. Spalton)

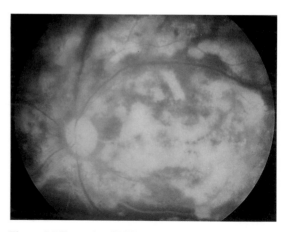

Figure 9.5 Extensive CMV retinitis (courtesy of Mr R. Marsh)

regional lymphadenopathy. The ulcer heals spontaneously during which time haematogenous spread has occurred leading to the secondary stage.

Secondary stage

The majority of the signs of secondary syphilis appear within the eighth week of infection although there may be considerable delay.

- Mucocutaneous involvement is usually the presenting feature. A macular, papular or mixed skin rash characteristically involving the palms and soles is common. Where the rash involves warm, moist areas such as the perianal region, the rash develops a warty appearance (condylomata lata). Mucous patches (snailtrack ulcers) may develop in the mouth and elsewhere. Occasionally the rash involves the eyelids and leaves a residual patchy skin depigmentation and alopecia of the eyelashes and eyebrows (madarosis). Patchy alopecia of the scalp also occurs.
- Systemic involvement may cause malaise, fever, generalized lymphadenopathy, meningitis, nephritis and hepatitis.

Latent stage

This follows resolution of secondary syphilis and can be detected only by serological tests.

Tertiary (late) stage

About 30% of untreated patients will progress to the tertiary stage within 5–30 years. However, some patients with tertiary syphilis have no memory of primary or secondary stages, and in some the signs may have been suppressed by antibiotics. The basic pathological lesion of tertiary syphilis is an area of tissue necrosis called a gumma, resulting from ischaemia, due to an obliterative endarteritis.

The main types of tertiary syphilis are:

- Cardiovascular giving rise to aortitis.
- Neurosyphilis which causes tabes dorsalis or general paralysis of the insane (GPI).
- Benign late syphilis characterized by gummata in tissues other than the cardiovascular system and CNS.

Syphilis and AIDS

Patients at risk from AIDS are also at risk from other sexually transmitted diseases, like syphilis, so that the two conditions may coexist. It appears that concomitant HIV infection may alter the natural course of syphilis, rendering the disease more aggressive with unusual manifestations. All patients with AIDS should therefore also be tested for syphilis and vice versa.

Diagnostic tests

VDRL (venereal disease research laboratory)   This is a non-specific reagin test which is useful for screening. If positive, one of the more specific tests below should be performed. The VDRL becomes positive shortly after the development of the primary chancre and becomes negative after adequate treatment. If it fails to do so, the course of antibiotics may have been only partially effective or patient compliance was poor. Further therapy should therefore be advised.

MHA-TP and TPHA (haemagglutination tests for Treponema pallidum)   These are useful specific tests for treponemal antibody but may be negative in early primary syphilis. They may also be positive in yaws.

FTA-ABS (fluorescent treponemal antibody absorption)   This is a specific test to detect antitreponemal antibodies. Once positive it remains positive throughout the patient's life despite treatment. However, the test is not titratable and is read as: reactive, weakly reactive or non-reactive.

Performing the VDRL and TPHA is an adequate screen in most cases.

Dark ground microscopic examination   This is performed on a chancre or mucocutaneous lesion for the presence of a spirochaete.

Ocular features

Ocular syphilis is rare and there are no pathognomonic signs. Eye involvement typically occurs during the secondary or tertiary stages.

External

Occasionally external features include: (1) scleritis, (2) interstitial keratitis and (3) madarosis.

Anterior uveitis

This occurs in about 4% of patients with secondary syphilis and is usually associated with the roseolar skin rash. Initially the uveitis is acute and unilateral. If untreated the fellow eye frequently becomes affected and the intraocular inflammation becomes chronic.

Choroiditis

- Multifocal choroiditis is the most common type and occurs typically during the late secondary stage. Active choroiditis is characterized by multiple grey-yellow lesions which are associated with a vitritis. Healed lesions appear as areas of chorioretinal atrophy associated with hyperpigmentation (see Figure 1.12).
- Unifocal choroiditis is less common and is frequently bilateral. It is characterized by an inflammatory focus near the disc (juxtapapillary choroiditis) or at the macula (central choroiditis).

Neuroretinitis

This consists of primary involvement of the retina and optic nerve, and is independent of choroidal inflammation. It occurs usually during the secondary stage and may be associated with meningitis. Unless treated, the retinal blood vessels become replaced by white strands, the optic disc becomes atrophic and areas of hyperpigmentation develop (Figure 9.6).

Neuro-ophthalmic lesions

Patients with neurosyphilis may develop:

- Pupillary abnormalities such as Argyll Robertson pupils.
- Ocular motor palsies of the third and sixth cranial nerves (see Chapter 6).
- Visual field defects due to gummatous involvement of the brain.

Treatment of ocular syphilis

- The patient should have a lumbar puncture to confirm neurosyphilis. If negative treat with aqueous procaine penicillin G 600 000 units (0.6 mega-units) intramuscularly daily for 15 days.
- If the CSF is abnormal 12 mega-units of penicillin G should be given intravenously for 10 days.

Penicillin-sensitive patients can be treated with tetracycline 500 mg four times a day for 30 days.

Congenital syphilis

Systemic features

The classic Hutchinson's triad of congenital syphilis is:

- Interstitial keratitis.
- Deafness.
- Typical changes of the teeth.

Other stigmata include: (1) rhagades, (2) sabre shin, (3) saddle nose and (4) Clutton's joints.

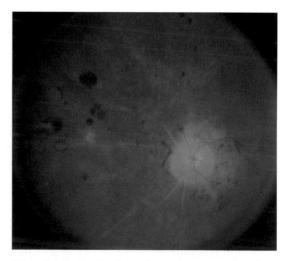

Figure 9.6 Optic atrophy and vascular attenuation due to old syphilitic retinitis

Ocular features

The two ocular manifestations are:

1. Interstitial keratitis.
2. Retinopathy:
   (a) finely pigmented peripheral 'salt and pep-
       per' type which is usually non-progressive
       and benign;
   (b) similar to retinitis pigmentosa.

Chlamydial oculogenital infection

Definition

Chlamydial oculogenital infection is a sexually
transmitted disease caused by serotypes D–K of
the organism *Chlamydia trachomatis*. Currently, it is
the most common sexually transmitted disease in
the UK and USA. It typically affects young adults
during their sexually active years.

Systemic features

- In men chlamydial infection is the most
  common cause of both 'non-specific urethritis'
  (NSU) and 'non-gonococcal urethritis' (NGU). It
  may also cause epididymitis, proctitis and it
  may act as a trigger for Reiter's disease (see
  Chapter 4).
- In women chlamydial infection may cause
  abacterial pyuria, cervicitis, proctitis, salpingitis, peritonitis and perihepatitis (Fitz–Hugh–
  Curtis syndrome). Chronic salpingitis may
  result in infertility.

Ocular features

In adults

- Conjunctivitis is usually bilateral, subacute and
  associated with a mucopurulent discharge and
  follicles in the fornices (Figure 9.7).
- Epithelial keratitis of the upper cornea is the
  most frequent corneal finding although marginal infiltrates (Figure 9.8) and a micropannus
  may also occur.

In infants

Chlamydia is a common cause of neonatal
conjunctivitis (ophthalmia neonatorum) as a result
of transfer of the organism from the mother's birth
canal. The eye infection typically develops between the fifth and fourteenth day after birth.

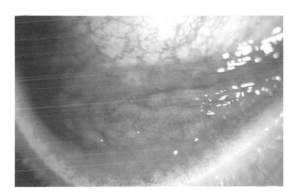

Figure 9.7 Chlamydial conjunctivitis with follicles in
inferior fornix

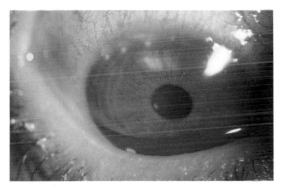

Figure 9.8 Superior marginal infiltrates in chlamydial
keratitis

Treatment

Adult infection

1. Topical tetracycline ointment four times a day for 6 weeks.
2. Systemic treatment can be with one of the following regimens:
   (a) oral oxytracycline or erythromycin 250 mg four times a day for 6 weeks or 500 mg four times a day for 1–2 weeks;
   (b) oral doxycycline 300 mg weekly for 3 weeks or 100 mg daily for 2 weeks.

Infantile infection

- Topical tetracycline.
- Systemic erythromycin 50 mg/kg in four divided doses before feeds for 2 weeks, or 3 weeks if there is associated chlamydial pneumonitis.

Gonorrhoea

Gonorrhoea is now a very rare cause of conjunctivitis. The infection is typically acute, severe and associated with a purulent discharge (Figure 9.9). Prompt diagnosis and treatment is essential because it may lead to corneal ulceration and perforation. The treatment is with intravenous aqueous penicillin G 10 mega-units a day for 5 days.

Further reading

BELIN, M.W., BALTCH, A.L. and HAY, P.B. (1981) Secondary syphilitic uveitis. *American Journal of Ophthalmology*, **92**, 210

CUHNA DE SOUZA, E.C., JALKH, A.E., TREMPE, C.L. *et al.* (1988) Unusual central chorioretinitis as the first manifestation of early secondary syphilis. *American Journal of Ophthalmology*, **105**, 271–276

HENDERLY, D.E., FREEMAN, W.R., CAUSEY, D.M. *et al.* (1987) Cytomegalovirus retinitis and response to therapy with ganciclovir. *Ophthalmology*, **94**, 425–434

KALINSKE, M. and LEONE, C.R. JR (1982) Kaposi's sarcoma involving eyelid and conjunctiva. *Annals of Ophthalmology*, **14**, 497–499

MORGAN, C.M., WEBB., R.M. and O'CONNOR, G.R. (1984) Atypical syphilitic chorioretinitis and vasculitis. *Retina*, **4**, 225

PASSO, M.S. and ROSENBAUM, J.T. (1988) Ocular syphilis in patients with human immunodeficiency virus infection. *American Journal of Ophthalmology*, **106**, 1–6

PEPOSE, J.S., NEWMAN, C., BACH, M.C. *et al.* (1987) Pathologic features of cytomegalovirus retinopathy after treatment with the antiviral agent ganciclovir. *Ophthalmology*, **94**, 414–424

ROSS, W.H. and SUTTON, H.F.S. (1980) Acquired syphilitic uveitis. *Archives of Ophthalmology*, **98**, 496–498

SCHUMA, J.S., ORELLANA, J., FRIEDMAN, A.H. *et al.* (1987) Acquired immunodeficiency syndrome (AIDS). *Survey of Ophthalmology*, **31**, 384–410

USSERY III, F.M., GIBSON, S.R., CONKLIN, R.H. *et al.* (1988) Intravitreal ganciclovir in the treatment of AIDS-associated cytomegalovirus retinitis. *Ophthalmology*, **95**, 640–648

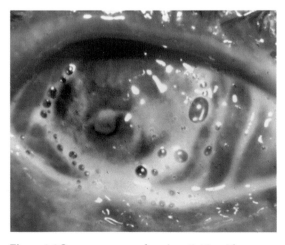

Figure 9.9 Severe gonococcal conjunctivitis with a purulent discharge

10

Skin disorders

Cicatricial pemphigoid

Definition

Cicatricial pemphigoid is a rare, idiopathic, chronic, progressive, autoimmune disease characterized by recurrent sub-basal blisters of the skin and mucous membranes. It affects women more commonly than men. Immunofluorescence shows IgG and C3 along the basement membrane and IgA deposition is sometimes observed.

Systemic features

Presentation is typically during late middle age.

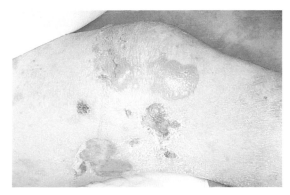

Figure 10.1 Bullous skin eruption in cicatricial pemphigoid

Skin

Skin lesions occur in about 25% of patients and are of two types:

1. Generalized bullous eruption, similar to pemphigoid but of shorter duration (Figure 10.1).
2. Localized erythematous plaques with recurrent vesicles and bullae affecting the scalp and skin near the affected mucous membranes. The lesions heal to leave smooth atrophic scars.

Mucous membranes

The oral mucosa is affected in 80% of cases. The mucous membranes of the nose, larynx, oesophagus, anus and vagina can also be involved. The submucosal blisters lead to erosions which may heal and leave scars and strictures.

Treatment

- Topical steroids alone may control localized skin lesions.
- Systemic steroids and azathioprine may be required for widespread disease.
- Dapsone may also be effective.

Ocular features

Essential shrinkage of the conjunctiva is a common and potentially very serious complication. Although involvement is always bilateral the disease is frequently asymmetrical with regard to time of onset, severity and rate of progression.

Signs

In chronological order:

- Subacute papillary conjunctivitis associated with a mucoid discharge is the presenting feature.
- Subconjunctival bullae form and, on bursting, give rise to conjunctival ulceration and the formation of pseudomembranes.
- Healing is associated with chronic inflammation, subepithelial fibrosis and conjunctival shrinkage.

Complications

- Dry eye due to fibrous occlusion of the ductules of the lacrimal and accessory lacrimal glands, as well as destruction of mucin-secreting conjunctival goblet cells.
- Symblepharon is a serious complication in which adhesions form between the palpebral and bulbar conjunctiva (Figure 10.2).
- Ankyloblepharon in which adhesions form at the outer canthi between the upper and lower eyelids.
- Eyelid deformities such as entropion (inturning of eyelids) and trichiasis (inturning of eyelashes).
- Corneal scarring secondary to ulceration, infection and vascularization may lead to blindness (Figure 10.3).

Treatment

- Systemic treatment is the same as for the skin and mucous membrane lesions.
- Local treatment includes steroids during the acute phase, artificial tears and surgery for severe structural complications.

Stevens–Johnson syndrome (severe bullous erythema multiforme)

Definitions

- Stevens–Johnson syndrome is a severe mucocutaneous disease caused by a hypersensitivity reaction to viruses, bacteria and drugs such as sulphonamides. In only 50% of cases is a cause found, herpes simplex and mycoplasma infections being the most common aetiological agents.
- Erythema multiforme is a milder condition presenting with peripheral lesions. The mucous membranes may or may not be affected.

Systemic features

Presentation

This is at any age with malaise, fever, sore mouth and possibly cough and arthralgia which may last for up to 14 days.

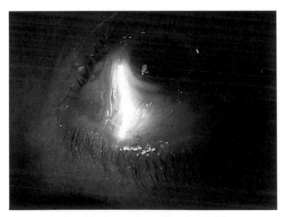

Figure 10.2 Symblepharon in ocular cicatricial pemphigoid

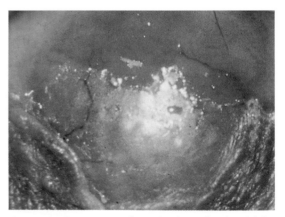

Figure 10.3 Severe corneal scarring in ocular cicatricial pemphigoid

Signs

In chronological order these are:

- The oral mucosa is always involved. Bullae produce erosions which, on the lips, lead to haemorrhagic crusting (Figure 10.4).
- Symmetrical, erythematous maculopapules, some of which develop into the target lesions (Figure 10.5).
- Vesiculobullous lesions which may become haemorrhagic.
- Healing occurs over 1–4 weeks and scarring may occur.

The disease may recur if the patient is re-exposed to the inciting agent.

Treatment

- Systemic steroids may be necessary in severe cases.
- Acyclovir is used if herpes simplex is suspected as the causative agent.

Ocular features

Signs

The conjunctiva is involved in 90% of cases. The signs in chronological order are:

- Mucopurulent papillary conjunctivitis (Figure 10.6).
- Focal red conjunctival infarcts form in ischaemic areas of the conjunctiva
- Yellow-white conjunctival membranes form, which, on shedding, leave focal fibrotic patches.

Early treatment with topical steroids may be beneficial.

Complications

- Conjunctival fibrosis and keratinization.
- Scarring of the eyelids.
- Aberrant eyelashes at the openings of the meibomian gland orifices (acquired distichiasis).
- Corneal scarring.

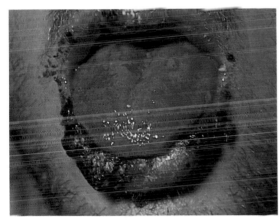

Figure 10.4 Haemorrhage crusting of lips in Stevens–Johnson syndrome

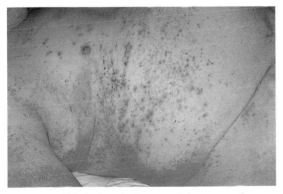

Figure 10.5 Skin lesions in Stevens–Johnson syndrome

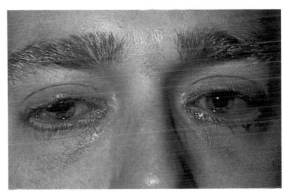

Figure 10.6 Severe conjunctivitis in Stevens–Johnson syndrome

- Corneal scarring and neovascularization is uncommon but it is the most frequent cause of visual morbidity.
- Posterior subcapsular cataracts are rare.
- Conical cornea (keratoconus) is also rare (Figure 10.11).

Treatment

- Eyelid hygiene, in the form of regular lid scrubs using a cotton bud dipped in a diluted solution of baby shampoo, is used to control the blepharitis.
- Topical steroids are the mainstay of treatment of conjunctivitis and keratitis, although topical sodium cromoglycate may also be useful.

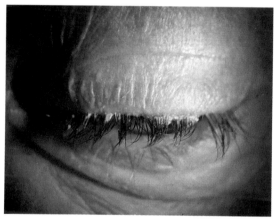

Figure 10.10 Staphylococcal blepharitis in patient with atopic eczema

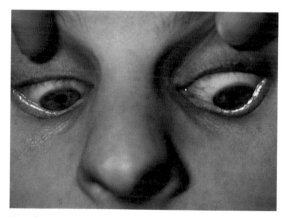

Figure 10.11 Bulging of the left lower eyelid due to keratoconus (Munson's sign)

Acne rosacea
Definition

Acne rosacea is a common idiopathic skin disorder affecting the convexities of the face. Persistent erythema leads to telangiectasia, and papules and pustules may be present. When it occurs, onset tends to be in the third to fourth decade.

Skin lesions

- Chronic hyperaemia of the face which typically involves the cheeks, forehead and nose, and produces the 'rosaceal complexion'. Flushing of affected areas of skin may be precipitated by alcohol, spicy foods, tea and coffee, or by changes in ambient temperature.
- Other features include variable degrees of telangiectasia, papules, pustules and hypertrophic sebaceous glands (Figure 10.12).
- Rhinophyma is the most advanced form of the disease.

Treatment

- Oral tetracycline reduces the number of papules and pustules. The initial dose is 250 mg four times a day for 1 month followed by 250 mg for at least 6 months (or twice a day throughout).

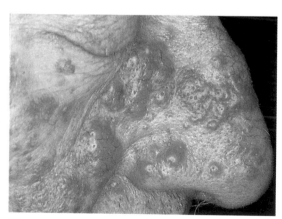

Figure 10.12 Hypertrophied sebaceous glands in severe acne rosacea

The antibiotic should be taken before meals but should not be given to pregnant women because of the risk of inducing discolouration of teeth in the offspring. The therapeutic effect of tetracycline does not appear to be related to its antibacterial action.

- Topical metronidazole is also useful.
- Avoidance of precipitating factors is helpful in reducing the severity of erythema.

Ocular features

Ocular complications are common and in some patients they antedate the skin lesions.

Signs

- Chronic seborrhoeic blepharitis is very common.
- Recurrent styes and meibomian cysts are also common.
- Peripheral keratitis is uncommon. It is characterized by peripheral vascularization especially involving the inferotemporal and inferonasal quadrants. Very rarely severe generalized corneal scarring and perforation may occur.

Treatment

- Topical steroids are a very effective short-term measure for keratitis, although long-term use may precipitate corneal melting.

- Systemic tetracycline is very useful for the ocular as well as the skin lesions.

Albinism

Definition

Albinism is a term applied to a group of rare genetically determined disorders of the melanin pigmentary system characterized by congenital hypopigmentation of hair, skin and eyes (oculocutaneous albinism) or limited to the eyes (ocular albinism). Oculocutaneous albinism is subdivided into the following two groups.

Complete albinism

These individuals are deficient in the enzyme tyrosinase and are incapable of synthesizing melanin. The clinical features are:

- Blonde hair (Figure 10.13) and fair skin.
- Diaphanous blue irides which are responsible for photophobia.
- Pendular nystagmus and grossly reduced visual acuity due to lack of differentiation of the fovea and hypopigmentation of the fundus (Figure 10.14).

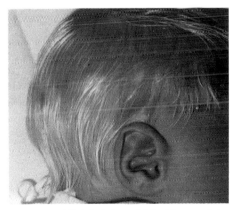

Figure 10.13 Fair hair in a child with complete albinism (courtesy of Dr R. Winter)

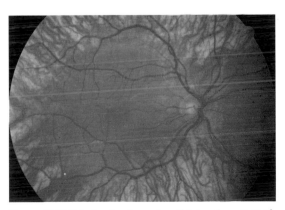

Figure 10.14 Pale fundus in ocular albinism (courtesy of Professor A. Fielder)

visual impairment due to optic atrophy may ensue. Pernicious anaemia may also cause dementia, peripheral neuropathy and subacute combined degeneration of the spinal cord characterized by posterior and lateral column disease.

Leukaemias

Definition

The leukaemias are a group of neoplastic disorders characterized by abnormal proliferation of white blood cells.

Systemic features

Acute leukaemias

The acute leukaemias typically present with anaemia, haemorrhage and infection, as well as with infiltration of the lymph nodes, spleen and liver.

- Acute lymphocytic leukaemia typically affects children. With appropriate chemotherapy the cure rate is about 60%.
- Acute myeloid leukaemia occurs more frequently in adults and has a much worse prognosis.

Chronic leukaemias

Chronic leukaemias typically affect the elderly and the presentation is usually more vague and gradual (e.g. fatigue, weight loss, infection). In some cases the diagnosis is made by chance. Chemotherapy often does not prolong survival although it may improve the quality of life.

Ocular features

Ocular involvement is more common in the acute than in chronic leukaemias. Virtually any or all of the ocular structures may be involved. It is, however, important to distinguish primary leukaemic infiltration, which is rare, from the more common secondary changes such as those due to associated anaemia, thrombocytopenia, hyperviscosity, opportunistic infections and the side effects of treatment (e.g. steroid-induced cataracts).

Anterior segment

Anterior segment disease is seen most frequently in patients with acute lymphocytic leukaemia. It is rare in patients with acute myeloid leukaemia and very rare in the chronic leukaemias. The main features are:

- Iritis and hypopyon – the most common.
- Iris thickening, either diffuse or nodular.
- Spontaneous subconjunctival haemorrhage (Figure 11.2).
- Spontaneous bleeding into the anterior chamber (hyphaema – Figure 11.3).

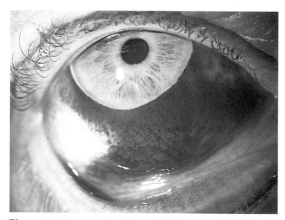

Figure 11.2 Large subconjunctival haemorrhage

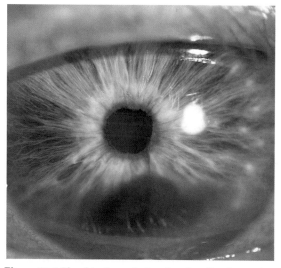

Figure 11.3 Blood in the anterior chamber (hyphaema)

Orbit

Orbital involvement is more common in acute than in chronic leukaemias, and it occurs more frequently in the lymphocytic then in the myeloid type. Orbital infiltration usually presents with painful proptosis, lid oedema and chemosis.

Retinopathy

Retinal involvement is common and is characterized by the following:

- Venous tortuosity and dilatation are early changes.
- Flame-shaped haemorrhages are usually located at the posterior pole and Roth's spots may also be present.
- Cotton-wool spots may be due to leukaemic infiltration or associated with anaemia or hyperviscosity.
- Peripheral retinal neovascularization is an occasional feature of chronic myeloid leukaemia.

Optic neuropathy

Infiltration of the optic nerve typically occurs in children with myeloid leukaemia and, unless promptly treated by radiotherapy, the risk of blindness is very high. Disc involvement is characterized by a fluffy infiltrate associated with variable disc oedema and haemorrhage (Figure 11.4). It is important to differentiate leukaemic optic neuropathy from papilloedema due to raised intracranial pressure secondary to meningeal infiltration.

Hyperviscosity syndromes

Definition

Hyperviscosity syndromes are a diverse group of rare disorders characterized by increased blood viscosity due to one of the following:

- Increased number of red cells in polycythaemia rubra vera and secondary polycythaemia.
- Increased number of white cells in the chronic leukaemias.
- Abnormal plasma proteins in Waldenström's macroglobulinaemia and rarely in multiple myeloma.

Ocular features

Retinal findings include venous dilatation, segmentation and tortuosity, as well as superficial and deep retinal haemorrhages, cotton-wool spots (Figure 11.5), retinal oedema, retinal vein occlusion and disc oedema.

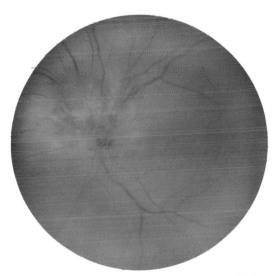

Figure 11.4 Infiltration of optic disc in acute myeloid leukaemia

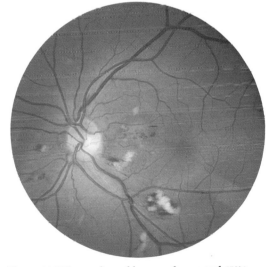

Figure 11.5 Flame-shaped haemorrhages and cotton-wool spots in polycythaemia rubra vera

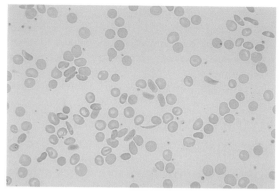

Figure 11.6 Blood film in sickle-cell anaemia showing sickling of erythrocytes (courtesy of Dr P. Mackie)

Sickle-cell disease

Pathogenesis

Sickling haemoglobinopathies are due to the presence of one, or a combination of, abnormal haemoglobins which cause the red blood cells to adopt an anomalous shape under conditions of hypoxia and acidosis (Figure 11.6). Because these deformed red blood cells are more rigid than normal cells, they may become impacted in, and obstruct, small blood vessels and cause tissue ischaemia with a marked local increase in acidosis and hypoxia, and even more sickling.

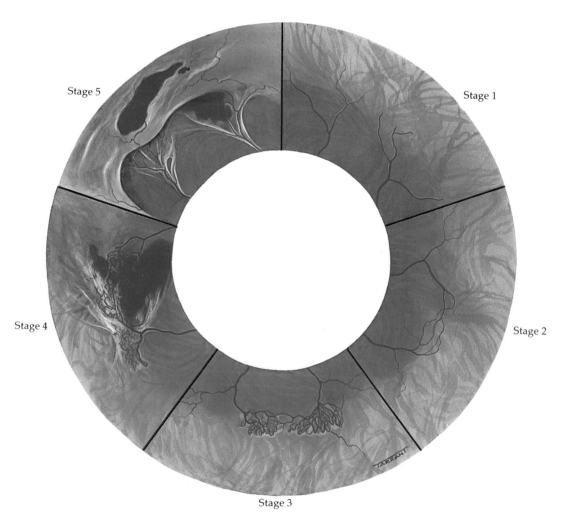

Figure 11.7 Progression of proliferative sickle-cell retinopathy

Abnormal haemoglobins

The sickling disorders in which the mutant haemoglobins S and C are inherited as alleles of normal haemoglobin A are of particular import-ance because of their ocular manifestations. These abnormal haemoglobins may occur in combination with normal haemoglobin A or in association with each other as follows:

- *AS* (sickle-cell trait) is present in 8% of American Blacks.
- *SS* or sickle-cell disease or sickle-cell anaemia which is present in 1% of American Blacks.
- *SC* or sickle-cell C disease which is present in 0.2% of American Blacks.
- *SThal* or sickle-cell thalassaemia.

Systemic features

- Sickle-cell trait (AS) is the mildest form and usually requires severe hypoxia or other abnor-mal conditions to produce sickling.
- SC and SThal are associated with mild anaemia but severe ocular complications.
- Sickle-cell disease (SS) causes severe systemic complications such as painful crises and severe haemolytic anaemia. Ocular complications, however, are usually mild and asymptomatic.

Ocular features

Proliferative sickle retinopathy

The most severe form of retinopathy occurs in SC and SThal. It can be divided into the following five stages (Figure 11.7).

Stage 1   This is characterized by peripheral arteriolar occlusion.

Stage 2   This shows peripheral arteriovenous anastomoses.

Stage 3   This is characterized by 'sea-fan' neovascularization from the anastomoses.

Stage 4   This is characterized by haemorrhage from the new vessels.

Stage 5   This is characterized by tractional retinal detachment.

Non-proliferative retinopathy

- Asymptomatic lesions are venous tortuosity, areas of peripheral chorioretinal atrophy (black sunbursts), peripheral pink superficial ('salmon patch') retinal haemorrhages, peripheral refrac-tive spots consisting of haemosiderin deposits, 'silver-wiring' of peripheral arterioles and, rarely, angioid streaks.
- Symptomatic lesions are caused by vascular occlusions.

Non-retinal manifestations

- Conjunctival isolated comma or corkscrew-shaped vascular segments.
- Ischaemic iris atrophy and occasionally rubeosis.

Further reading

FOULDS, W.S. (1987) 50th Bowman Lecture. 'Blood is thicker than water'. Some haemorheological aspects of ocular disease. *Eye*, **1**, 343–363

HOOVER, D.L., SMITH, L.E., TURNER, S.J. *et al.* (1988) Ophthalmic evaluation of survivors of acute lymphob-lastic leukemia. *Ophthalmology*, **95**, 151–155

KINCAID, M.C. and GREEN, W.R. (1983) Ocular and orbital involvement in leukemia. *Survey of Ophthalmology*, **27**, 211–232

LEVEILLE, A.S. and MORSE, P.H. (1981) Platelet-induced retinal neovascularization in leukemia. *American Jour-nal of Ophthalmology*, **91**, 640–643

NOVAKOVIC, P., KELLIE, S.J. and TAYLOR, D. (1988) Child-hood leukaemia: relapse in the anterior segment. *British Journal of Ophthalmology*, **73**, 354–359

ROSENTHAL, A.R. (1983) Ocular manifestations of leu-kemia: a review. *Ophthalmology*, **90**, 899–905

RUBINFELD, R.S., GOOTENBERG, J.E., CHAVIS, R.M. *et al.* (1988) Early onset acute orbital involvement in childhood lymphoblastic leukemia. *Ophthalmology*, **95**, 116–120

SARNAT, R.L. and JAMPOL, L.M. (1986) Hyperviscosity retinopathy secondary to polyclonal gammopathy in patients with rheumatoid arthritis. *Ophthalmology*, **93**, 124–127

SCHACHAT, A.P., MARKOWITZ, J.A., GUYER, D.R. *et al.* (1989) Ophthalmic manifestations of leukemia. *Archives of Ophthalmology*, **107**, 697–700

THOMAS, D.J. (1983) Haematological aspects of cerebral arterial disease. In: R.W.Ross Russell (Ed.) *Vascular Disease of the Central Nervous System*, pp. 337–355. Edinburgh: Churchill Livingstone

12

Malignant diseases

Metastatic carcinoma

Choroidal metastases

Primary sites

The breast is the most common primary site in females and the bronchus in males. A choroidal secondary may be the initial presentation of a bronchial carcinoma, whereas a past history of mastectomy is the rule in patients with breast metastases. Other less common primary sites include the kidney, testis and gastrointestinal tract. The prostate is, however, an extremely rare primary site.

Clinical features

Although choroidal metastases may occur anywhere in the fundus, they have a definite predilection for the posterior pole.

- Typically they appear as solitary or multiple, creamy-white, placoid or oval lesions with ill-defined borders (Figure 12.1). Bilateral involvement is frequent. Secondary exudative retinal detachment is a common complication.
- Rarely the metastases invade the optic nerve head and cause a severe loss of vision (Figure 12.2).

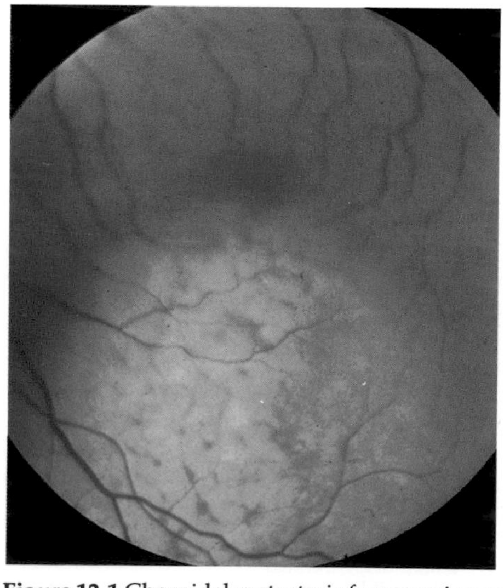

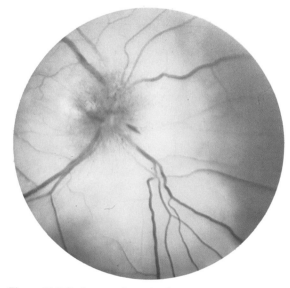

Figure 12.1 Choroidal metastasis from a primary breast carcinoma (courtesy of Mr T. ffytche)

Figure 12.2 Optic nerve invasion by metastatic carcinoma

Orbital metastases

Primary sites

Excluding leukaemia and lymphoma, breast carcinoma and lung carcinoma are the most frequent sources of orbital metastases, followed by the prostate. It is common for the orbital metastasis to antedate the discovery of the primary tumour.

Clinical features

Orbital metastases usually present with subacute proptosis, pain, diplopia, eyelid swelling, ptosis, a red eye, watering and decreased vision.

Leptomeningeal metastases

Primary sites

Tumours of the breast, bronchus and skin melanomas are the most common primary sites that metastasize to the leptomeninges. Occasionally meningeal involvement occurs before the primary tumour is discovered.

Clinical features

Meningeal carcinomatosis is notoriously difficult to diagnose. In the early stages the patient may merely complain of mild visual loss and isolated non-specific symptoms such as headache. Later features are severe visual impairment due to damage to the optic nerve and diplopia due to ocular motor cranial nerve involvement. However, in many cases the correct diagnosis depends on a meticulous cytological study of the CSF.

Multiple myeloma

Definition

Multiple myeloma is a rare neoplasm of plasma cells that are derived from B lymphocytes (Figure 12.3).

Systemic features

Presentation is usually in late adult life with weakness, anorexia and weight loss. More advanced cases may present with renal failure, anaemia, infection or bone involvement.

- Abnormal monoclonal protein (M protein) is present in the blood, urine, or both. Free light chains (Bence Jones protein) may also be present in the urine.
- Lytic punched-out lesions in red marrow-bearing bones (skull, spine, ribs, proximal extremities and pelvis) consisting of focal collections of plasma cells are common (Figure 12.4). They cause pain and may lead to

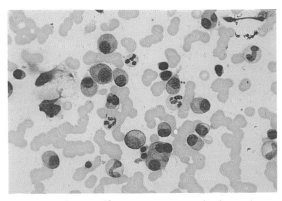

Figure 12.3 Smear of bone marrow in myltiple myeloma (courtesy of Dr P. Mackie)

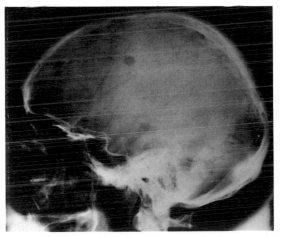

Figure 12.4 Lytic skull lesions in multiple myeloma (courtesy of Dr J.M. Stevens)

pathological fractures. Vertebral fractures may cause spinal cord or nerve root injury.

- Generalized osteoporosis due to diffuse demineralization.
- Proteinuria is very common. Renal damage is caused by infiltration of the kidney by myeloma, hypercalcaemia, toxic effects of light chains on the tubules and amyloid deposition.
- Neurological involvement may occur due to nerve compression by fractures, encephalopathy associated with hyperviscosity or peripheral nerve infiltration by amyloid.
- Hypercalcaemia.

Treatment

Treatment is with alkylating agents (melphalan, cyclophosphamide) and systemic steroids. Radiotherapy may be useful in treating plasmacytomas and localized lytic bone lesions. The prognosis is poor with a mean survival rate of 2–3 years.

Ocular features

- Corneal involvement with fine crystalline deposits is uncommon and usually innocuous.
- Cysts of the ciliary epithelium filled with proteinaceous fluid are very common. They are invariably asymptomatic and are rarely detected during life.
- Retinopathy consisting of flame-shaped haemorrhages, haemorrhages with white centres (Roth's spots) and cotton-wool spots is common. The retinopathy associated with hyperviscosity is, however, rare.
- Orbital plasmacytomas, either arising in the soft tissues or in the surrounding bones with secondary orbital invasion, are rare. They often respond to local irradiation.

Lymphomas
Definition

Lymphomas are a group of malignant disorders that primarily affect the lymphatic system. The two main types are: (1) Hodgkin's disease and (2) non-Hodgkin's lymphomas.

Systemic features

Presentation has two peaks: between the ages of 15 and 30 and after the age of 50 years.

- Asymptomatic swelling of lymph nodes is the most frequent presenting feature.
- Systemic symptoms such as fever and weight loss are common in Hodgkin's disease and in high grade non-Hodgkin's lymphomas.

Patients who are immunosuppressed (e.g. renal transplants, AIDS) are at increased risk of non-Hodgkin's lymphomas.

Treatment

Treatment according to the stage, is with radiotherapy, chemotherapy or both. The prognosis is variable.

Ocular features

Intraocular involvement

This is extremely rare except in reticulum cell sarcoma which is a highly malignant multicentric form of non-Hodgkin's (large cell histiocytic) lymphoma. The two main forms are the systemic and the less common central nervous system type. The systemic type primarily involves the lymph nodes, visceral organs and, rarely, the uveal tract. The CNS type primarily involves the central nervous system and also frequently the eye. Ocular findings may precede CNS involvement by months or even years. Both eyes are eventually affected in 80% of cases, but the severity of involvement is frequently asymmetrical. Ocular reticulum cell sarcoma should be suspected in the following circumstances:

- Chronic anterior uveitis unresponsive to steroids.
- Chronic vitritis (intermediate uveitis) in an elderly patient. Vitreous biopsy may be useful for cytological confirmation.
- Subretinal infiltration with yellowish, multifocal, solid, subretinal lesions with hyperpigmented spots, is virtually pathognomonic (Figure 12.5). Exudative retinal detachment is a rare and late complication.

Treatment of both CNS and ocular reticulum cell sarcoma is with radiotherapy.

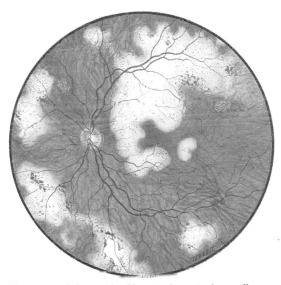

Figure 12.5 Subretinal infiltration by reticulum cell sarcoma

Orbit

The orbit is involved in about 1% of patients with systemic lymphomas. In most cases orbital involvement, which may be bilateral, is usually a late feature of the disease and does not present any diagnostic problems (Figure 12.6). However, diagnostic difficulties may be occasionally encountered in patients with orbital lymphomas who have no clinical evidence of systemic disease. Although histological differentiation between inflammatory orbital pseudotumours and frank malignant lymphomas is usually easy, in a few cases the histological features raise suspicion of malignancy and yet the lesion resolves spontaneously or with the help of systemic steroids. In other patients, what looks like a benign reactive lymphoid hyperplasia localized to the orbit may be followed several years later by the development of a systemic lymphoma.

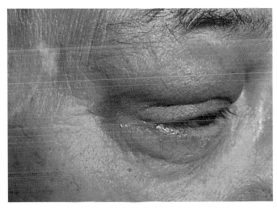

Figure 12.6 Orbital lymphoma

Conjunctiva

Conjunctival involvement (Figure 12.7) is common in non-Hodgkin's lymphomas but very rare in Hodgkin's disease.

Further reading

BOLDT, H.C. and NERAD, J.A. (1988) Orbital metastases from prostate carcinoma. *Archives of Ophthalmology*, **106**, 1403–1408

CANTILLO, R., JAIN, J., SINGHAKOWINTA, A. *et al.* (1979) Blindness as an initial manifestation of meningeal carcinomatosis in breast cancer. *Cancer*, **44**, 755–757

CARRIERE, V.M., KARCIOGLU, Z.A., APPLE, D.J. *et al.* (1982) A case of prostatic carcinoma with bilateral orbital metastases and the review of the literature. *Ophthalmology*, **89**, 402–406

CHAR, D.H., LJUNG, B-M., MILLER, T. *et al.* (1988) Primary intraocular lymphoma (ocular reticulum cell sarcoma). Diagnosis and management. *Ophthalmology*, **95**, 625–630

FREEDMAN, M.I. and FOLK, J.C. (1987) Metastatic tumours to the eye and orbit: Patient survival and clinical characteristics. *Archives of Ophthalmology*, **105**, 1215–1219

FREEMAN, L.N., SCHACHAT, A.P., KNOX, D.L. *et al.* (1987) Clinical features, laboratory investigations, and survival in ocular reticulum cell sarcoma. *Ophthalmology*, **94**, 1631–1639

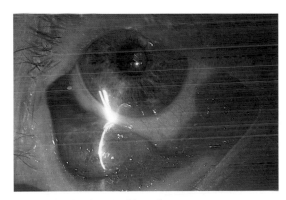

Figure 12.7 Conjunctival lymphoma

GROSSNIKLAUS, H.E., FARHI, D.C., JACOBSON, B.R. *et al.* (1988) Malignant lymphoma of the conjunctiva following Hodgkin's disease. *British Journal of Ophthalmology*, **72**, 212–215

HORNBLASS, A., KASS, L.G. and REICH, R. (1987) Thyroid carcinoma metastatic to the orbit. *Ophthalmology*, **94**, 1004–1007

KIRMANI, M.H., THOMAS, E.L. RAO, N.A. *et al.* (1987) Intraocular reticulum cell sarcoma: diagnosis by choroidal biopsy. *British Journal of Ophthalmology*, **71**, 748–752

KNAPP, A.J., GARTNER, S. and HENKIND, P. (1987) Multiple myeloma and its ocular manifestations. *Survey of Ophthalmology*, **31**, 343–351

McCRARY III, J.A., PATRINELY, J.R. and FONT, R.L. (1986) Progressive blindness caused by metastatic occult signet-ring gastric carcinoma. *Archives of Ophthalmology*, **104**, 410–413

MEWIS, L. and YOUNG, S.E. (1982) Breast carcinoma metastatic to the choroid. *Ophthalmology*, **89**, 147–151

NELSON, C.C., HERTZBERG, B.S. and KLINTWORTH, G.K. (1983) A histopathologic study of 716 unselected eyes in patients with cancer at the time of death. *American Journal of Ophthalmology*, **95**, 788–793

SIEGEL, M.J., DALTON, J., FRIEDMAN, A.H. *et al.* (1989) Ten-year experince with primary ocular 'reticulum cell sarcoma' (large cell non-Hodgkin's lymphoma. *British Journal of Ophthalmology*, **73**, 342–346

WEISENTHAL, R., FRAYER, W.C., NICHOLS, C.W. *et al.* (1988) Bilateral ocular disease as the initial presentation of malignant lymphoma. *British Journal of Ophthalmology*, **72**, 248–252

13

Phacomatoses

Definition

The phacomatoses are a group of uncommon conditions characterized by the presence of hamartomas involving various organs such as the skin, eye, central nervous system and viscera.

Sturge–Weber syndrome

Systemic features

The Sturge–Weber syndrome (*encephalotrigeminal angiomatosis*) is the only phacomatosis without a hereditary tendency.

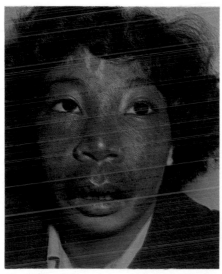

Figure 13.1 Bilateral naevus flammeus in Sturge–Weber syndrome. Note facial hypertrophy of the involved area

Facial skin capillary angioma

A facial angioma (naevus flammeus) is present at birth and roughly involves the area of distribution of the first and/or second divisions of the trigeminal nerve. The skin lesion may be associated with hypertrophy of the involved area of the face (Figure 13.1). Occasionally the angioma extends across the midline and may even involve the upper trunk and upper arms.

Central nervous system

An ipsilateral angioma of the meninges and brain, which most frequently involves the parieto-occipital region, is common. The brain lesion may cause jacksonian-type epilepsy, hemiparesis and hemianopia. Atrophy of the neighbouring cerebral cortex may lead to variable degrees of mental handicap. The intracranial lesion frequently calcifies and can be detected by plain skull X-rays but is more obvious on MRI or CT scanning

Ocular features

Ocular manifestations are very common and consist of:

- Diffuse unilateral choroidal haemangioma (Figure 13.2).
- Haemangiomas of the episclera, iris and ciliary body.
- Glaucoma which occurs in 30% of cases and may cause a large eye (buphthalmos).

Neurofibromatosis

Systemic features

The neurofibromatoses are a group of hereditary disorders that primarily affect the cell growth of neural tissues. Inheritance is an autosomal dominant trait with irregular penetrance and variable expressivity. The mutation rate is high. The three main types are:

1. *Neurofibromatosis 1* (peripheral form) which is the most common.
2. *Neurofibromatosis 2* (central form) mainly consisting of bilateral acoustic neuromas with few if any cutaneous findings.
3. *Segmental* where features of the peripheral form are confined to one segment of the body.

Neural tumours

Tumours may occur of the brain, spinal cord, meninges, cranial nerves, peripheral nerves, sympathetic nerves, auditory nerve (acoustic neuroma) and adrenal gland (phaeochromocytoma).

Bone defects

Congenital bony defects may involve the greater wing of the sphenoid bone which may cause a pulsating proptosis, and occasional defects in the vertebrae and long bones. Some patients also have facial hemiatrophy (Figure 13.3).

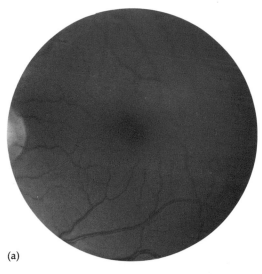

(a)

(b)

Figure 13.2 (a) Diffuse choroidal haemangioma in a patient with the Sturge–Weber syndrome; (b) fellow normal eye for comparison. (Courtesy of P.H. Morse)

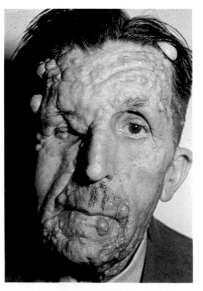

Figure 13.3 Right facial hemiatrophy in a patient with severe neurofibromatosis

Skin lesions

- Café-au-lait spots are flat light-brown patches which vary in size from a few millimetres to several centimetres (Figure 13.4). They appear at or soon after birth and increase in size and number throughout childhood. Some patients develop axillary freckling, a clinical sign unique to the disease.

- Fibromata mollusca are pedunculated, flabby, pigmented nodules which are frequently widely distributed over the body (Figure 13.5).
- Cutaneous plexiform neurofibromata consisting of enlarged peripheral nerves begin to appear at about puberty and increase in number throughout life. On palpation they resemble a bag of worms.

Ocular features

- Melanocytic, bilateral, iris hamartomas (Lisch nodules) are universal after the age of 16 years. The nodules have a smooth outline and are dome shaped (Figure 13.6).
- Choroidal hamartomas are present in about 30% of cases. They appear as discrete flat or slightly elevated areas of hyperpigmentation, dark brown-black in colour.
- Eyelid neuromas may give rise to a mechanical ptosis associated with a characteristic S-shaped deformity (Figure 13.7).
- Glioma of the optic nerve typically presents between the ages of 4 and 8 years with a gradual onset of unilateral proptosis and visual impairment. The optic disc may show either atrophy

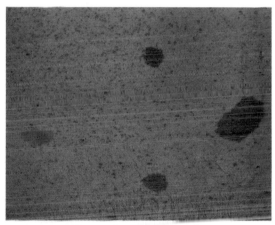

Figure 13.4 Café-au-lait patches in neurofibromatosis

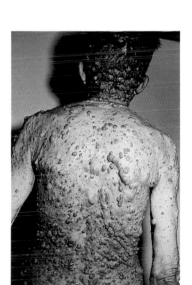

Figure 13.5 Fibroma molluscum in severe neurofibromatosis

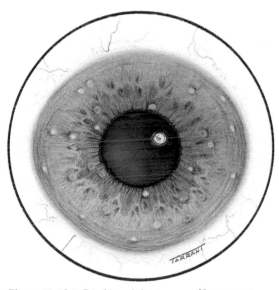

Figure 13.6 Iris (Lisch) nodules in neurofibromatosis

or oedema. In about 90% of patients, the tumour involves the anterior aspect of the optic canal and causes an enlargement of the optic foramen. Ultrasonography and CT show an enlargement of the optic nerve (Figure 13.8).

- Spheno-orbital encephalocele, caused by a congenital defect in the sphenoid bone, may give rise to a pulsatile congenital proptosis which is not associated with either a bruit or a thrill.
- Glaucoma is uncommon and, when present, this is at birth and is frequently associated with an ipsilateral lid neurofibroma.
- Prominent corneal nerves.
- Orbital plexiform neuroma.
- Congenital ectropion uveae.

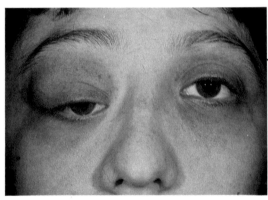

Figure 13.7 Mechanical ptosis due to a neurofibroma of right upper eyelid

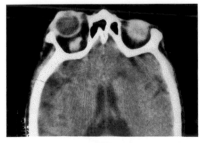

Figure 13.8 CT scan showing enlargement of the optic nerve due to an optic nerve glioma

Tuberous sclerosis

Systemic features

Tuberous sclerosis (Bourneville's disease) is inherited as an autosomal dominant trait, although 50% of cases represent new mutations.

Skin lesions

- Nodular fibroangiomas ('adenoma sebaceum') are vascularized red papules which have a butterfly distribution around the nose and cheeks (Figure 13.9a). These lesions are inconspicuous at birth, but they slowly multiply and enlarge and become clinically obvious between the ages of 2 and 5 years. On cursory examination they may be mistaken for acne vulgaris, hence the term 'adenoma sebaceum'.
- Achromic naevi, consisting of hypopigmented patches involving the trunk, limbs and scalp, are pathognomonic of tuberous sclerosis (Figure 13.9b). In infants with little skin pigmentation these lesions may only be detected under ultraviolet light (Wood's lamp) as fluorescent patches.

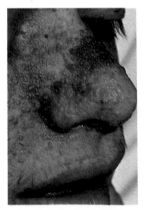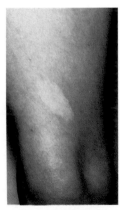

Figure 13.9 Tuberous sclerosis. (a) Severe adenoma sebaceum; (b) achromic naevus of thigh (courtesy of Dr R. Winter)

- Café-au-lait spots similar to those seen in patients with neurofibromatosis may represent late hyperpigmentation of achromic naevi.
- Shagreen patches consist of diffuse fibrous thickenings over the lumbar region.

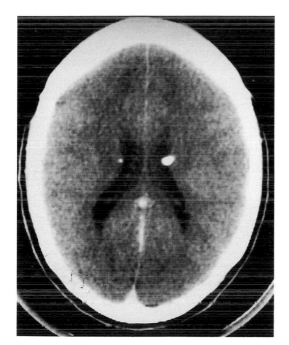

Figure 13.10 CT scan showing subependymal calcified hamartomas in tuberous sclerosis (courtesy of Dr J.M. Stevens)

Central nervous system

Slowly growing astrocytic hamartomas of the central nervous system are a universal finding. Although they may be found anywhere in the brain they tend to concentrate in a periventricular area (Figure 13.10). Complications of the hamartomas include:

- Epilepsy in 80%.
- Mental handicap in 60%.
- Hydrocephalus due to blockage of CSF circulation is uncommon.
- Malignant transformation – very rare.

Visceral hamartomas

These lesions are usually asymptomatic and may involve the kidneys and heart (rhabdomyomas), as well as other organs and the subungual areas (Figure 13.11).

Ocular features

- Fundus astrocytomas are present in about 50% of patients. These benign tumours, which are bilateral in 15% of cases, may be single or multiple and are most frequently situated at or near the optic nerve head (Figure 13.12). Early tumours are small and semitranslucent. Later they become more opaque and the development of calcification within the tumours may

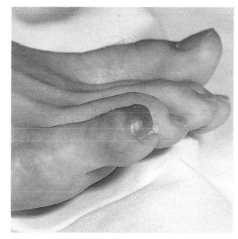

Figure 13.11 Subungual hamartoma in tuberous sclerosis

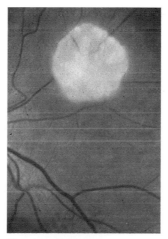

Figure 13.12 Retinal astrocytoma in tuberous sclerosis (courtesy of Mr T. ffytche)

give them a mulberry-like appearance (Figure 13.13). Treatment is unnecessary because they are asymptomatic and innocuous.

- Hypopigmented iris spots are common.
- Hypopigmented fundus lesions are uncommon.

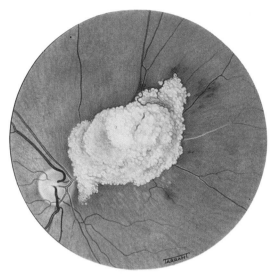

Figure 13.13 Large mulberry-like retinal astrocytoma in tuberous sclerosis

Von Hippel–Lindau syndrome

Systemic features

The von Hippel–Lindau syndrome is inherited as an autosomal dominant trait with incomplete penetrance and delayed expressivity. Usually the following systemic features become manifest after the onset of ocular symptoms.

Central nervous system

The most frequent systemic presentation is with neurological dysfunction caused by haemangioblastomas which may involve the cerebellum, medulla, pons and spinal cord.

Miscellaneous

- Cysts of the kidneys, pancreas, liver, epididymis, ovary and lungs.
- Hypernephroma and phaeochromocytoma.
- Polycythaemia.

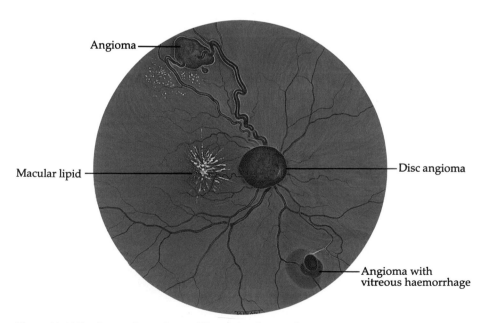

Figure 13.14 Fundus angiomas in von Hippel–Lindau syndrome

Ocular features

The only ocular manifestations are capillary haemangiomas of the retina and optic nerve head (Figure 13.14), which may be multiple and are bilateral in 50% of cases. However, only about 25% of patients with fundus tumours have systemic involvement. Because it is impossible to predict which patients with ocular lesions will have systemic tumours, it is essential to refer all for a thorough systemic and neurological evaluation. Relatives should also be screened in view of the dominant mode of inheritance of this condition. The early lesions are small red nodules which then grow into larger orange-red tumours. Arteriovenous shunting within the tumour gives rise to dilatation and tortuosity of its associated artery and vein, so that both vessels appear similar in colour. Angiomas of the optic disc are not associated with abnormal vessels. Complications of retinal angiomas are the following:

- Hard exudates due to chronic leakage of plasma from the tumour inevitably develop in untreated cases. The exudates not only form in the area surrounding the tumour but also in remote areas of the fundus. Deposition of hard exudates at the macula will have a profound effect on visual acuity.
- Exudative retinal detachment and bleeding are late complications.

All tumours are vision threatening and should be treated. The various treatment modalities include photocoagulation, cryotherapy and penetrating diathermy.

Ataxia telangiectasia (Louis–Bar syndrome)

Systemic features

Ataxia telangiectasia is inherited as an autosomal recessive trait and is characterized by:

- Progressive cerebellar ataxia becoming clinically apparent in early childhood.
- Cutaneous telangiectasia involving the ears, face, lips and extensor surfaces of both extremities.
- Mental handicap which becomes apparent at adolescence.

Ocular features

- Telangiectasia of the bulbar conjunctiva typically develops between the ages of 4 and 7 years (Figure 13.15).
- Ocular motility defects include oculomotor apraxia, fixation nystagmus, strabismus and poor convergence.

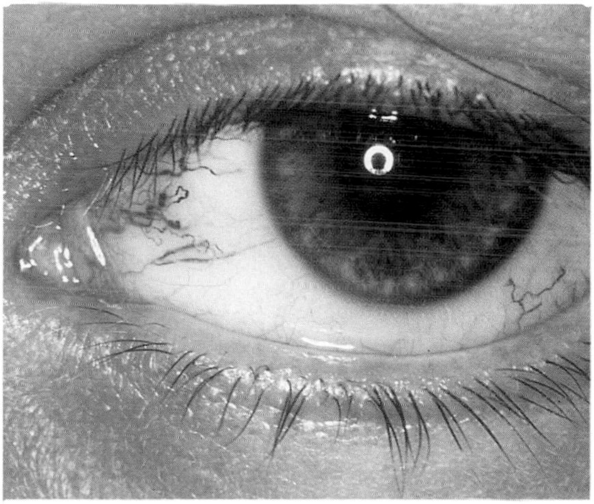

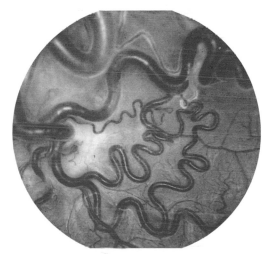

Figure 13.15 Telangiectasia of bulbar conjunctiva in Louis–Bar syndrome

Figure 13.16 Retinal racemose haemangioma in Wyburn–Mason syndrome (courtesy of Professor A.C. Bird)

Wyburn–Mason syndrome

This consists of racemose haemangiomas of the midbrain and of the retina (Figure 13.16).

Further reading

COTLIER, E. (1977) Café au lait spots in the fundus in neurofibromatosis. *Archives of Ophthalmology*, **95**, 1990–1992

HUSON, S., JONES, D. and BECK,L. (1987) Ophthalmic manifestations of neurofibromatosis. *British Journal of Ophthalmology*, **71**, 235–238

LEWIS, R.A. and RICCARDI, V.M. (1981) von Recklinghausen's neurofibromatosis. Incidence of iris hamartomas. *Ophthalmology*, **88**, 348–354

PERRY, H.D. and FONT, R.L. (1982) Iris nodules in von Recklinghausen's neurofibromatosis. Electron microscopic confirmation of their melanocytic origin. *Archives of Ophthalmology*, **100**, 1635–1640

WILLIAMS, R. and TAYLOR, D. (1985) Tuberous sclerosis. *Survey of Ophthalmology*, **30**, 143–154

14

Miscellaneous disorders

Systemic associations of ectopia lentis

Marfan's syndrome

Definition

Marfan's syndrome is a dominantly inherited widespread abnormality of connective tissue.

Systemic features

Cardiac

- Aortic incompetence, dilated aortic root, coarctation of the aorta, mitral incompetence with a floppy valve and dissecting aortic aneurysm. Death may occur during the mid-forties.

- Bacterial endocarditis may occur even in the presence of mild cardiac anomalies.

Skeletal

- The limbs are disproportionately long as compared with the trunk (Figure 14.1).
- Long spider-like fingers and toes (arachnodactyly) (Figure 14.2).
- Funnel or pigeon chest.
- Hyperextensibility and instability of joints.
- Flat feet, kyphoscoliosis and a high arched palate.

Miscellaneous

- Muscular underdevelopment, hernias and decrease in subcutaneous fat.

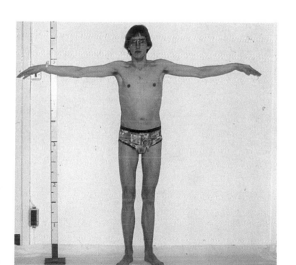

Figure 14.1 Marfan's syndrome

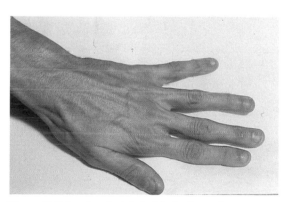

Figure 14.2 Arachnodactyly in Marfan's syndrome

143

- Cystic lung disease which may cause spontaneous pneumothorax.
- Small papules in the skin of the neck (Miescher's elastoma).

Ocular features

- Lens subluxation which is upward, bilateral and non-progressive is present in about 70% of cases (Figure 14.3). It is associated with a tremulous iris (iridodonesis).
- Microspherophakia (small and spherical lens) is present in some cases (Figure 14.4).
- Glaucoma may be associated with lens subluxation or an angle anomaly.
- Hypoplasia of dilator pupillae makes the pupil difficult to dilate.
- Flat cornea (cornea plana).
- Myopia (Figure 14.5) and retinal detachment (Figure 14.6).

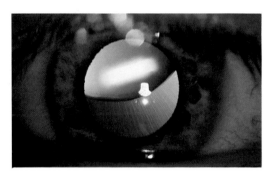

Figure 14.3 Upward lens subluxation in Marfan's syndrome

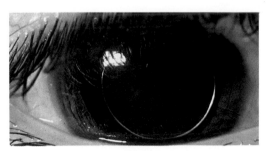

Figure 14.4 Microspherophakia

Homocystinuria

Definition

Homocystinuria is a rare, recessively inherited disorder of methionine metabolism due to a deficiency of cystathione-β-synthetase. It is the second most common inborn error of amino acid

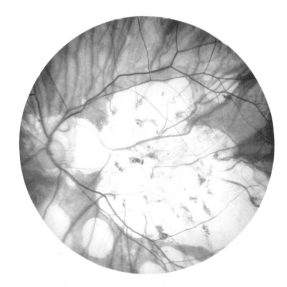

Figure 14.5 Severe myopic degeneration

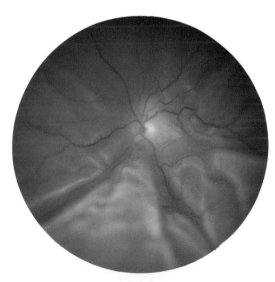

Figure 14.6 Total retinal detachment

metabolism. Plasma homocysteine is increased, chiefly as the disulphide homocystine (homocysteine–homocysteine), and spills into the urine. Plasma methionine is likewise increased and plasma cysteine and cystine are decreased. The mechanism by which the biochemical abnormalities produce the clinical features have not been fully explained.

Systemic features

There are no characteristic features in infancy and early detection relies on screening of the urine of newborn babies. The clinical diagnosis may be difficult because the age of onset, severity and pattern manifestations vary widely. The typical untreated homocystinuric is asymptomatic in infancy and subsequently develops ectopia lentis, mental handicap, skeletal disorders and life-threatening thromboembolic episodes.

- Increased platelet stickiness occurs which may predispose to thrombosis, particularly following general anaesthesia.
- Skeletal anomalies include arachnodactyly, osteoporosis and fractures.
- Miscellaneous features include mental handicap, fine hair and a malar flush.

Homocystine levels vary widely and tests based on methionine loading may confirm the diagnosis in suspected cases missed on routine screening.

Treatment

One form of homocystinuria responds to pyridoxine (vitamin B$_6$), the other more common and more severe form is pyridoxine unresponsive and requires a low-methionine diet supplemented with cystine. The risk of ocular complications can be substantially reduced in patients started on treatment within 6 weeks of birth.

Ocular features

- Lens subluxation is bilateral and usually downwards with complete disruption of the zonules. It occurs in up to 70% of patients by the age of 8 years and in more than 95% by 40 years.
- Glaucoma may occur either due to pupil block or dislocation of the lens into the anterior chamber (Figure 14.7).

Ehlers–Danlos syndrome

Definition

This is a rare, usually dominantly inherited, disorder of collagen caused by deficiency of hydroxylysine.

Systemic features

- Skin is thin, hyperextensible (Figure 14.8) and heals poorly.

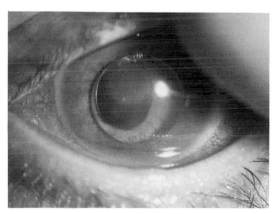

Figure 14.7 Dislocation of a microspherophakic lens into the anterior chamber in homocystinuria

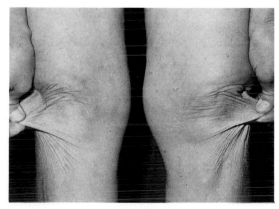

Figure 14.8 Skin hyperelasticity in Ehlers–Danlos syndrome (courtesy of Dr R. Pope)

- Hyperextensibility of joints (Figure 14.9) which may be associated with recurrent dislocation, repeated falls, hydrarthrosis and pseudotumour formation over the knees and elbows.
- Kyphoscoliosis, genu recurvatum and flat feet are also frequent.
- Bleeding diathesis.
- Dissecting aneurysms and spontaneous rupture of large blood vessels.
- Mitral valve prolapse.
- Diaphragmatic hernias and diverticula of the gastrointestinal and respiratory tracts.

Ocular features

- *Common*: epicanthic folds, conical cornea (keratoconus – see Figure 10.11), high myopia, retinal detachment and angioid streaks (see Figure 10.9).
- *Uncommon*: blue sclera and lens subluxation.

Systemic associations of retinitis pigmentosa

Definition of retinitis pigmentosa

Retinitis pigmentosa is a generic name for a group of inherited diseases characterized by night blindness and constricted visual fields. The clinical features of retinitis pigmentosa vary between patients, and even among family members with the disease.

Clinical features

Presentation

This is usually during the second decade with night blindness.

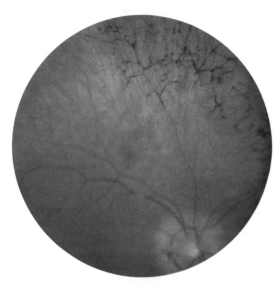

Figure 14.10 'Bone-spicule' pigmentation in retinitis pigmentosa

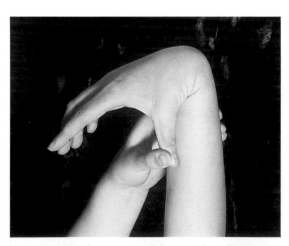

Figure 14.9 Joint hyperextensibility in Ehlers–Danlos syndrome (courtesy of Dr A. Hall)

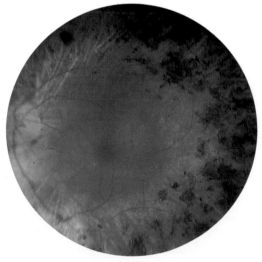

Figure 14.11 Advanced retinitis pigmentosa with unmasking of choroidal vessels

Signs

- Peripheral retina shows perivascular 'bone-spicule' pigmentation and arteriolar attenuation (Figure 14.10), and later unmasking of the larger choroidal blood vessels (Figure 14.11).
- Optic disc is initially normal but later becomes waxy pale.
- Maculopathy may be cystoid, atrophic or cellophane.
- Associations include open-angle glaucoma, posterior subcapsular cataracts, myopia and occasionally conical cornea (keratoconus).

Systemic associations

Retinitis pigmentosa, often of the atypical type, may be associated with the following systemic diseases.

Bassen–Kornzweig syndrome (abetalipoproteinaemia)

This disease typically affects Ashkenazi Jews and is inherited as an autosomal rescessive trait. It is characterized by:

- Fat malabsorption from birth.
- Spinocerebellar ataxia.
- Acanthocytosis.
- Abetalipoproteinaemia.

The disease is ultimately fatal although treatment with vitamins A and E may be beneficial in some cases.

Refsum's syndrome (phytanic acid storage disease)

This disease is inherited as an autosomal recessive trait. It is characterized by:

- Hypertrophic peripheral neuropathy.
- Cerebellar ataxia.
- Elevated CSF protein in the absence of pleocytosis (cytoalbuminous inversion).
- Deafness.
- Ichthyosis.

Treatment with a phytanic acid-free diet and plasma exchange may prevent progression of both the systemic and ocular lesions.

Usher's syndrome

This recessively inherited disorder is characterized by congenital, non-progressive, sensorineural deafness. Usher's syndrome accounts for about 5% of all cases of profound deafness in children and is responsible for about half of all cases of combined deafness and blindness. Another important cause of combined congenital deafness and blindness is maternal rubella.

Kearns–Sayre syndrome

This consists of a triad of:

- Chronic progressive external ophthalmoplegia (ocular myopathy) (see Chapter 6).
- Heart block that may cause sudden death.
- Retinitis pigmentosa.

The Kearns–Sayre syndrome usually becomes manifest prior to the age of 20 years and in some cases it is associated with short stature, delayed puberty, mental handicap, cerebellar ataxia and deafness.

Laurence–Moon–Biedl syndrome

This recessively inherited disorder is characterized by:

- Mental handicap.
- Polydactyly and syndactyly.
- Hypogonadism.
- Obesity.

Friedreich's ataxia

This recessively inherited disorder is characterized by:

- Posterior column disease.
- Ataxia.
- Nystagmus.

Mucopolysaccharidoses
Definition

The mucopolysaccharidoses (MPS) are a group of rare inborn errors of metabolism involving zymes that metabolize basic compounds of connective tissue. There are six major MPSs some of which have more than one phenotype.

Systemic features

The main features are skeletal anomalies, mental handicap and facial coarseness (Figure 14.12).

Ocular features

- Corneal deposition occurs in all MPSs, except Hunter's and Sanfilippo's. It is most severe in Hurler's and Scheie's and causes corneal clouding which is present at birth. In general corneal changes are associated with skeletal anomalies.

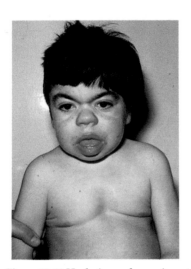

Figure 14.12 Hurler's syndrome (courtesy of Dr R. Winter)

- Pigmentary retinopathy may occur in all MPSs, apart from Morquio's and Maroteaux–Lamy. In general it is associated with mental handicap.
- Optic atrophy has been reported in all six MPSs.

The ocular changes are summarized in Table 14.1 below.

Retinopathy of prematurity
Definition

Retinopathy of prematurity (ROP) is a rare proliferative retinopathy which typically affects premature infants exposed to high ambient oxygen concentrations. Infants who weigh less than 1300 g are at particular risk.

Clinical features

Although ROP is a bilateral condition, the severity of involvement in the two eyes is frequently asymmetrical. The active stage of the disease is divided into the following five stages:

Stage 1

Demarcation line consists of a thin tortuous white line parallel with the ora serrata which separates the avascular immature retina from the vascularized retina (Figure 14.13a).

Stage 2

The line develops into a ridge containing isolated neovascular tufts (Figure 14.13b).

Table 14.1 Ocular changes in the mucopolysaccharidoses

		Corneal deposits	Retinopathy	Optic atrophy
MPS 1-H	= Hurler	+++	+	+
MPS 1-S	= Scheie	+++	+	+
MPS 2	= Hunter	–	+	+
MPS 3	= Sanfilippo	–	+	+
MPS 4	= Morquio	+	–	+
MPS 6	= Maroteaux–Lamy	+	–	+

Stage 3

The ridge is associated with fibrovascular proliferation which may cause vitreous haemorrhage (Figure 14.13c).

Stage 4

Subtotal tractional retinal detachment typically develops about 10 weeks after birth (Figure 14.13d).

Stage 5

Total tractional retinal detachment.

Spontaneous regression occurs in about 80% of cases, even from stage 3.

Screening

Who to screen

All infants born at less than 36 weeks or who weigh less than 2000 g who have received supplemental oxygen should be screened.

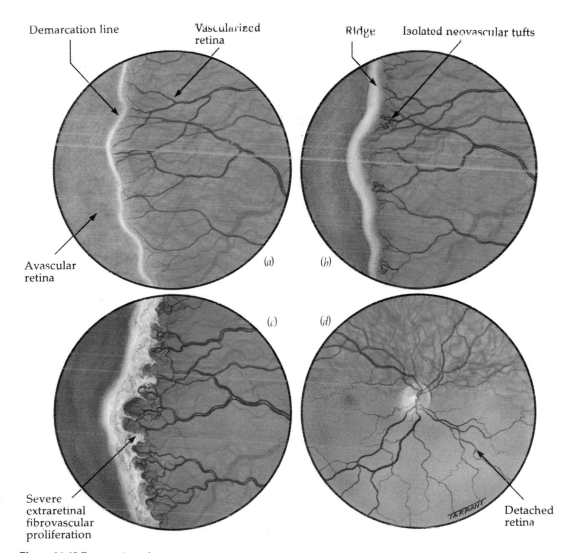

Figure 14.13 Progression of active retinopathy of prematurity

When to screen

Screening during the first month of life is of limited value because the pupils are frequently difficult to dilate and visualization of the fundus is impaired by vitreous haze. The most useful time to screen is between the seventh and ninth weeks of life. This is because ROP rarely appears for the first time after 9 weeks, and retinal detachment seldom develops before that time.

How to screen.

The pupils of premature infants should be dilated with a combination of cyclopentolate 0.5% and phenylephrine 2.5%. The retina should then be examined with an indirect ophthalmoscope and any abnormalities carefully documented.

Treatment

At present there is no treatment for active ROP that is universally accepted. This is partly due to the difficulty in evaluating results because of the high rate of spontaneous regression. The following therapeutic measures have been advocated:

- Cryotherapy to ablate the immature avascular peripheral retina.
- Vitreoretinal surgery for tractional retinal detachment (stage 5).
- Vitamin E is of uncertain value. It has been suggested that vitamin E deficiency may be a

contributing factor in the development of ROP. However, the administration of vitamin E may cause undesirable systemic side effects and at present the risks vs benefits are unclear.

Further reading

BURKE, J.P., O'KEEFE, M., BOWELL, R. *et al.* (1989) Ocular complications in homocystinuria – early and late treated. *British Journal of Ophthalmology*, **73**, 427–431

COGAN, D.G., RODRIGUES, M., CHU, F.C. *et al.* (1984) Ocular abnormalities in abetalipoproteinaemia. *Ophthalmology*, **91**, 991–998

COMMITTEE FOR THE CLASSIFICATION OF RETINOPATHY OF PREMATURITY (1984) An international classification of retinopathy of prematurity. *Archives of Ophthalmology*, **102**, 1130–1134

FISHMAN, G.A., KUMAR, A., JOSEPH, M.E. *et al.* (1983) Usher's syndrome. *Archives of Ophthalmology*, **101**, 1367–1374

McKECHNIE, N.M., KING, M. and LEE, W.R. (1985) Retinal pathology in the Kearns–Sayre syndrome. *British Journal of Ophthalmology*, **69**, 63–75

PALMER, E.A. (1981) Optimal timing of examination of acute retrolental fibroplasia. *Ophthalmology*, **88**, 662–666

PATZ, A. (1985) Observations on the retinopathy of prematurity. *American Journal of Ophthalmology*, **100**, 164–168

SCHAFFER, D.B., JOHNSON, L., QUINN, G.E. *et al.* (1985) Vitamin E and retinopathy of prematurity. *Ophthalmology*, **92**, 1005–1011

TASMAN, W. (1985) Management of retinopathy of prematurity. *Ophthalmology*, **92**, 995–999

15

Ocular toxicity from systemic drugs

Systemic steroids

Uses

Systemic steroids are used in a wide variety of diseases. The two main indications are (1) suppression of a disease process (e.g. asthma, systemic lupus erythematosus, sarcoidosis), and (2) replacement therapy following hypophysectomy or adrenalectomy.

Ocular side effects

By far the most common ocular side effect of systemic steroid administration is the formation of lens opacities (cataract). The other less important complication is steroid-induced glaucoma.

Steroid cataract

Incidence The exact relationship between the total dose, weekly dose and duration of administration of steroids, and the risk of cataract formation is unclear. Earlier studies showed that cataract developed only in patients receiving moderate or high maintenance doses for longer than 1 year. Patients receiving less than 10 mg/day of prednisone equivalent or those treated for less than 1 year were considered immune. However, it is now apparent that some patients may develop lens opacities after short-term therapy and that cataract formation is not inevitable following prolonged administration. On this basis it has been suggested that the concept of a 'safe' dose should be abandoned, although the risk of cataract

formation appears to be less with alternate-day than with daily administration.

Clinical features Steroid-induced lens changes start as vacuoles which turn into opacities in the posterior subcapsular part of the lens (Figure 15.1a). Opacities then develop in the anterior subcapsular region (Figure 15.1b) and if steroid therapy is continued the entire lens may become opaque and the pupil white (mature cataract). Screening for cataract is easy and does not require the services of an ophthalmologist (see Chapter 1).

Management If possible, patients with steroid-induced cataracts should have their steroid therapy reduced to a minimum consistent with the control of the disease or changed to alternate-day therapy. Regression of early opacities may occur when the drug is stopped or reduced although progression may occur despite withdrawal. Patients with severe lens opacities will need to be referred to an ophthalmic surgeon. In the absence of other serious eye pathology, the results of surgery are excellent.

Steroid-induced glaucoma

Whilst the prolonged use of strong topical steroids (e.g. dexamethasone, betamethasone) causes an elevation of intraocular pressure in about 30% of the general population the propensity of systemic steroids to elevate intraocular pressure is very much less. It is therefore unnecessary for patients on systemic steroids to have their intraocular pressures measured at regular intervals by an ophthalmologist.

Antimalarials

Uses

The antimalarial drugs chloroquine (Nivaquine, Avlocor) and hydroxychloroquine (Plaquenil) are used in the prophylaxis and treatment of malaria as well as in the treatment of certain rheumatological (e.g. rheumatoid arthritis, juvenile chronic arthritis, systemic lupus erythematosus) and dermatological diseases (e.g. discoid lupus). The use of chloroquine has also been advocated in the treatment of calcium abnormalities of sarcoidosis. The normal adult daily dose in the treatment of rheumatological disorders is 250 mg of chloroquine phosphate or equivalent.

Ocular side effects

The two main ocular side effects of antimalarials are retinal damage and corneal deposits. Although uncommon, the retinal changes are potentially serious, and the corneal changes, which are extremely common, are innocuous.

Maculopathy

Incidence   The incidence of retinal damage is dose related. A cumulative dose of less than 100 g of chloroquine or a duration of treatment of less than 1 year is rarely associated with retinal damage. The risk of toxicity increases significantly when the additive dose exceeds 300 g (i.e. 250 mg daily for 3 years). However, there have been reports of patients receiving cumulative doses exceeding 1000 g who did not develop maculopathy. Hydroxychloroquine appears to be safer than chloroquine. The incidence of retinotoxicity is lower and, when retinal damage does occur, it is usually mild and non-progressive.

Clinical features   Chloroquine maculopathy can be divided into the following stages:

- Premaculopathy is characterized by normal visual acuity, and a scotoma to a red target between 4° and 9° of fixation. The changes usually disappear if the drug is stopped.
- Established maculopathy is characterized by slightly reduced visual acuity, loss of the foveolar reflex and a subtle parafoveal halo of

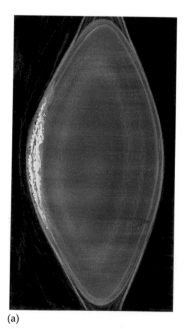 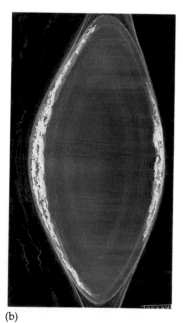

(a)   (b)

Figure 15.1 Progression of steroid-induced cataract: (a) early posterior subcapsular opacities; (b) posterior and anterior opacities

retinal pigment epithelial pallor (Figure 15.2a and Figure 15.3a). These changes are usually non-progressive if the drug is stopped.

- Bull's eye maculopathy is characterized by moderately reduced visual acuity, central foveolar hyperpigmentation surrounded by a depigmented zone and encircled by a hyperpigmented ring (Figures 15.2b, 15.3b). This stage may progress even if the drug is stopped.

- Severe maculopathy is characterized by marked reduction of visual acuity and a 'pseudo-hole' at the fovea with widespread surrounding retinal pigment epithelial atrophy (Figure 15.2c).

- End-stage maculopathy is characterized by severe reduction of visual acuity and marked atrophy of the retinal pigment epithelium with unmasking of the larger choroidal blood vessels (Figure 15.2d). The retinal arterioles may also

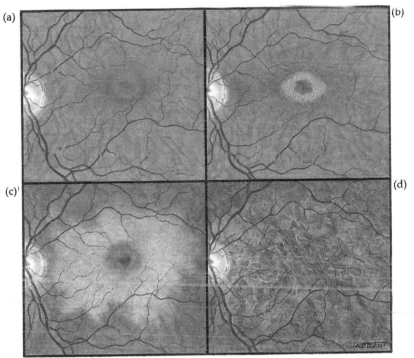

Figure 15.2 Progression of chloroquine maculopathy

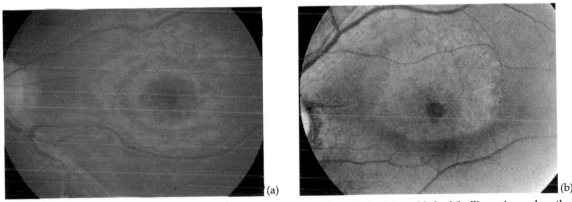

Figure 15.3 Chloroquine maculopathy: (a) early changes with a parafoveal halo; (b) established 'bull's-eye' maculopathy

become attenuated and pigment clumps develop in the peripheral retina. These changes are irreversible.

Screening At present there is no single test that is sufficiently reliable to rule out early maculopathy. However, in clinical practice chloroquine can be administered safely to patients without the need for repetitive routine examination by an ophthalmologist or the use of complicated tests. Recording of visual acuity and ophthalmoscopy by the prescribing doctor is all that is required to detect early maculopathy. If an abnormality is found then the opinion of an ophthalmologist should be sought.

Keratopathy

Chloroquine keratopathy is due to the deposition of the drug in the corneal epithelium, but unlike chloroquine maculopathy, it is not dose related. The changes are usually reversible on cessation of therapy, although occasionally they may disappear despite continued administration. In the vast majority of cases the keratopathy is innocuous, although very rarely it may cause symptoms of haloes and slight visual impairment. Unless gross, chloroquine keratopathy can only be detected by using a special microscope (slit lamp). The corneal changes consist of bilateral and symmetrical greyish or golden deposits in the superficial corneal epithelium that appear in a vortex fashion from a point below the pupil and swirl outwards (vortex keratopathy, cornea verticillata) (Figure 15.4).

Amiodarone

Uses

Amiodarone (Cardarone) is used mainly in the treatment of ventricular and supraventricular tachycardias including the Wolff–Parkinson–White syndrome.

Ocular side effects

- Keratopathy is identical to that seen with chloroquine but is dose related. On a low dose of 100–200 mg/day very mild changes may develop in some patients. On higher doses of 400–1400 mg/day a moderate to severe keratopathy occurs depending on the duration of administration. The corneal changes are reversible when the drug is stopped.
- Lens opacities, which are visually inconsequential, develop in about 50% of patients on moderate to high doses.

Chlorpromazine

Uses

Chlorpromazine (Largactil) is widely used as a sedative and in the treatment of schizophrenia. The normal maintenance oral dose is 75–300 mg/day.

Ocular side effects

- Retinotoxicity may occur but only if extremely high doses (over 2400 mg/day) are taken over long periods of time.
- Fine yellowish-brown granules may develop on the anterior lens surface. These are initially situated within the pupillary area but are rarely sufficiently dense to impair vision.

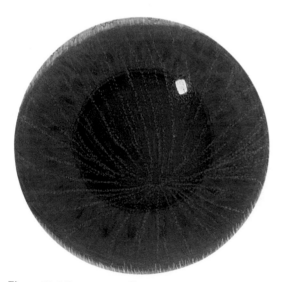

Figure 15.4 Cornea verticillata

Thioridazine

Uses

Thioridazine (Melleril) is used in the treatment of schizophrenia and related psychoses. The normal dose is 150–600 mg/day.

Ocular side effects

Retinotoxicity may develop when a daily dose of 800 mg is exceeded. Contrary to chloroquine maculopathy, the incidence of toxicity is unrelated to the total cumulative dose. The most characteristic symptoms of early toxicity are blurring of vision and impaired night vision or dark adaptation.

- Early changes are characterized by coarse, brownish pigmentary stippling at the posterior pole. Cessation of the drug at this stage may halt further damage.
- Late changes consist of geographical areas of atrophy and hyperpigmented clumps and plaques (Figure 15.5).

Tamoxifen

Uses

Tamoxifen (Emblon, Noltam, Nolvadex, Tomofen) is a specific antioestrogen used in the treatment of breast cancer. It has few systemic side effects and ocular complications are uncommon. The normal dose is 20–40 mg/day.

Ocular side effects

- Retinotoxicity in the form of multiple paramacular refractile lesions may develop in some patients on high doses. The retinal lesions, if severe, may cause visual impairment (Figure 15.6). The lowest cumulative dose reported to cause retinal changes is 7.7 g.
- Vortex keratopathy occurs in some patients.
- Bilateral optic neuritis, which is reversible on cessation of therapy, has been reported in a few cases.

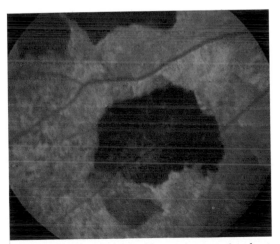

Figure 15.5 Clumps of retinal hyperpigmentation due to thioridazine toxicity (courtesy of Professor A. Bird)

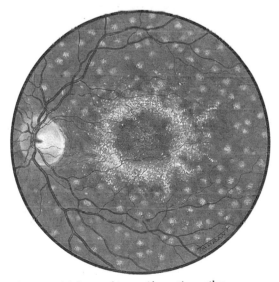

Figure 15.6 Advanced tamoxifen retinopathy

Ethambutol

Uses

Ethambutol (Myambutol, Mynah) is used in combination with isoniazid or rifampicin in the treatment of tuberculosis. The normal dose is 25 mg/kg per day for the first 2 months and 15 mg/kg per day thereafter.

Ocular side effects

About 1% of patients develop optic neuropathy on a dose of 15 mg/kg per day. The risk is increased with higher doses, particularly in patients with impaired renal function. Visual loss is usually sudden and dramatic with impairment of colour perception especially to red/green.

- The optic discs may either be normal or they may show oedema and splinter-shaped haemorrhages.
- Although a variety of visual field defects may occur the most common is a temporal defect.

Recovery is the rule once the drug is stopped, although this is frequently very slow and may take up to 12 months. Unfortunately, there is no test that can identify patients who will develop optic neuropathy. Ideally, a baseline examination should be performed before treatment is commenced. If the daily dose exceeds 15 mg/kg screening at 4-weekly intervals is recommended, particularly in patients with impaired renal function. The patient should be advised to stop taking the drug immediately he develops visual symptoms.

Further reading

ASHFORD, A.R., DONEV, R.P. and GARRETT, T.J. (1988) Reversible ocular toxicity related to tamoxifen therapy. *Cancer*, **61**, 33–35

CRUESS, A.F., SCHACHAT, A.P., NICHOLL, J. *et al.* (1985) Chloroquine retinopathy. Is fluorescein angiography necessary? *Ophthalmology*, **92**, 1127–1129

EHRENFELD, M., NESHER, R. and MERIN, S. (1986) Delayed-onset chloroquine retinopathy. *British Journal of Ophthalmology*, **70**, 281–283

FLECK, B.W., BELL, A.L., MITCHELL, J.D. *et al.* (1985) Screening for antimalarial maculopathy in rheumatology clinics. *British Medical Journal*, **291**, 782–785

JOHNSON, M.W. and VINE, A.K. (1987) Hydroxychloroquine therapy in massive doses without retinal toxicity. *American Journal of Ophthalmology*, **104**, 139–144

KAISER-KUPFER, M.I., KUPFER, C. and RODRIGUES M.M. (1981) Tamoxifen retinopathy. A clinicopathologic report. *Ophthalmology*, **88**, 89–93

McKEOWN, C.A., SWARTZ, M., BLOM, J. *et al.* (1981) Tamoxifen retinopathy. *British Journal of Ophthalmology*, **65**, 177–179

PUGESGAARD, T. and VON EYBEN, F.E. (1986) Bilateral optic neuritis evolved during tamoxifen treatment. *Cancer*, **58**, 383–386

Index